12/8/01

Eric —

you have been one of the corn[...]

of our Center. Whatever h[...]

I am ever so appreciat[...]

and right action. Joy and [...]

you — Kenn

ALTERNATIVE
HEALING
SECRETS

ALTERNATIVE HEALING SECRETS

AN A-TO-Z GUIDE TO ALTERNATIVE THERAPIES

MARIAH JAGER

Foreword by Dian Dincin Buchman, Ph.D.

GRAMERCY BOOKS
New York

This 1998 edition is published by Gramercy Books,®
a division of Random House Value Publishing, Inc.,
201 E. 50th Street, New York, NY 10022,
under arrangement with Ottenheimer Publishers, Inc.
5 Park Center Court, Suite 300, Owings Mills, MD 21117
SH140M L K J I H G F E D C B A

Gramercy Books® and colophon are registered trademarks of
Random House Value Publishing, Inc.

Random House
New York • Toronto • London • Sydney • Auckland
http://www.randomhouse.com/

Printed and bound in the United States of America.

Library of Congress Cataloging-in-Publication Data,
Jager, Mariah, 1969–
     Alternative healing secrets : an a-to-z guide to alternative therapies /
Mariah Jager; foreword by Dian Dincin Buchman.
          p.   cm.
     1. Alternative medicine—Popular works. I. Buchman, Dian Dincin.
II. Title.
R733.J27 1998
615.5—dc21   97-52140
ISBN 0-517-16047-1   CIP

                         8 7 6 5 4 3 2 1

This is for "Little Bear." Thanks for making it possible.

NOTE TO THE READER

The information in *Alternative Healing Secrets* is designed to increase your knowledge of healing practices that may relieve some conditions. This book is intended for use as a reference resource only, and not as a substitute for proper and prompt medical care. Use this volume to complement, not to replace, any treatment or advice your physician may prescribe or recommend. For best results, seek your physician's approval before using any of the methods or remedies that are listed in this book.

TABLE
OF
CONTENTS

FOREWORD

By Dian Dincin Buchman, Ph.D.

The other night while listening to a BBC radio feature, I was captivated by the smooth-as-silk voice of Prince Charles as he petitioned the British medical establishment to include more alternative medicine in the British health system. "The prince believes in, and uses a great many complementary medicines," the moderator explained. The prince was followed by several interesting interviews with average people who also regularly use alternative healing methods. One young woman with a serious case of psoriasis explained that her choice stemmed from dissatisfaction with the orthodox medical approach to her disease. "Fortunately, now I'm taking acupuncture and Chinese herbal treatments . . . . For the first time in my life I have a glimmer of hope," she said.

For many, this glimmer has turned into a bright shining ray. Several years ago, Harvard Medical School researchers reported that one-third of the American population is seeking health solutions from alternative medicine. Dr. David Eisenberg, the key spokesman for the study, suggested that the tendency towards "unconventional" treatments increased when patients could not find answers to perplexing personal health problems. He speculated it was only common sense for the public to ask the question, "What else can I do to get better?" In increasing numbers, people are turning to alternative health care to both supplement and complement their physician's advice, and it is a trend that is here to stay.

What does alternative medicine mean? Simply put, it includes those healing methods not generally accepted into mainstream medicine. Many are based on the wisdom of ages, using tried-and-true remedies and therapies dating back to ancient times. Some are the norm in other lands, but have yet to be embraced by our Western culture. Some can be done easily at home, for little or no expense. Almost all look for links between the mind and body, and how the body works as a whole with interdependent systems and functions. Alternative therapies also tend to be preventive in nature, or are geared toward eradicating the source of disease, rather than treating individual flare-ups of conditions. Let me share some personal examples.

Like millions of other Americans, I choose to take nutritional supplements every day to bolster my general health and overcome specific health problems. But oddly, despite clear evidence from meticulous research, nutrition or diet therapy is not yet a part of mainstream medical care! I visit my chiropractor, not only to manipulate and restore my often aching back, but on a monthly—sometimes even weekly—preventive basis. I practice herbal therapy for sleep, energy, and first aid, and serve herbal teas during meals to aid digestion. Each day, each week, each month, I use any number of easy, safe, no-cost, water therapy techniques. Cold water treading increases my resistance to disease. Drinking two glasses of cold water upon awakening prevents constipation, and a nightly hot bath ensures a good night's sleep. Other simple remedies I use in the privacy of my own home include mustard foot baths to prevent congestion, and cold compresses to produce instant internal heat and promote healing. My home medicine chest includes favorite tissue salts, a Bach flower Rescue Remedy, and an increasingly diverse list of homeopathic remedies. The list goes on.

A few insurance plans are beginning to cover alternative health care, but most such therapies are out-of-pocket expenses. I strongly feel the results justify the costs.

Does this mean I do all my own doctoring? No. For checkups and for maintaining my overall health I also go to a wonderful board-certified internist who shares my interest in holistic medicine. My doctor understands that health is a dynamic condition, and that it means much more than the mere absence of disease.

What does all this mean for you, the reader? Knowledge is power. *Alternative Healing Secrets* is an informative, on-target source book. It demystifies the jargon and practices used in alternative medicine, including those I have mentioned here. Because it is balanced and objective, you can trust that the author is not trying to "sell" any particular method at the risk of your health. Instead, the book provides valuable historical and scientific background on many alternative therapies so that you can gain control over your own health decisions and make educated choices that are right for you. Think of this volume as a starting point in your exploration of alternative healing, and then turn to the list of resources included in each section for more information.

Here's to your health!

Dian Dincin Buchman, Ph.D.
New York

Dian Dincin Buchman, who holds a doctorate in Health Sciences, is the author of several books on health and beauty, including *Herbal Medicine, The Complete Guide to Natural Sleep, The ABC's of Natural Beauty, The Complete Herbal Guide to Natural Health and Beauty, The Complete Book of Water Therapy,* and *Ancient Healing Secrets.*

INTRODUCTION

If you've broken your arm, sprained your ankle, or been in a car wreck, there's no better place to go than the emergency room. Today's Western doctors are second to none at putting your body back together after an emergency.

But what if you have chronic fatigue? Or persistent back pain? Or dozens of other conditions that modern medicine can still do little for?

In the past, you wouldn't have had much choice of treatment methods. You'd see your family "doc," who might give you some tests, prescribe some pills, and tell you to get plenty of rest. Now, after decades of not getting much healthier while paying more and more in medical bills, some folks are asking for an alternative—alternative medicine. Thanks to increasing interest in therapies to try in place of or along with standard Western health care, there are now scores of alternative kinds of health care in this country. Ranging from the old, like Ayurveda, to the new, like biofeedback, there are more options to choose from than ever before when you're looking to treat any number of common conditions that continue to resist modern medicine.

Besides gaining popular momentum, alternative (sometimes called "complementary") therapies are also starting to gain respect. The National Institutes of Health has established the Office of Alternative Medicine to investigate the effectiveness of many alternative therapies. And some major medical insurers—notorious for being ultraconservative—will even reimburse you for certain alternative treatments, like acupuncture, when they find the evidence is convincing enough to warrant it.

As you'll find, exploring alternative medicine is largely about taking charge of your own well-being. Similar to the benefits you reap from controlling stress, exercising, eating well, and taking your vitamins and minerals, alternative medicine offers a blend of care that treats not just your body, but your mind and spirit as well.

This book will help you explore today's most common alternative therapies. Chapters describe the history of each therapy, what it can and cannot treat, and what to expect when you seek that specific type of alternative care. Whenever possible we have included information on associated costs. And when necessary, we've also included a warning feature, called Alternative Alert, that explain any risks you may encounter with that therapy as well as when it's time to consult your family physician.

Enjoy it in good health.

ACUPUNCTURE
AND
ACUPRESSURE

Five-Thousand-Year-Old "Modern Medicine"

Two of the most well-known and well-accepted alternative healing practices are also two of the oldest. Both practices hail from the Far East, and both are based on a belief that we have certain points on our bodies that, when stimulated, have the power to heal.

ACUPUNCTURE: HEALING TO THE POINT

It is one of the most commonly prescribed treatments for addiction. Around the world, people insist that it relieves chronic pain. And it's quickly gaining popularity in the United States. Some remarkable new wonder drug? No. It's an ages-old old remedy that's as common in Asian countries as taking two aspirin is here in the West. It is acupuncture, and since its introduction into the American mainstream some thirty years ago, the practice has grown by leaps and bounds. Currently, nine to twelve million acupuncture treatments are performed in the United States each year.

A healing practice that originated in China, acupuncture is based on the belief that health is determined by a balanced, harmonious flow of vital life energy, known as *qi* (also spelled ki or chi and pronounced "chee"), throughout the body. According to this system, qi travels through your body

1

along fourteen major pathways, which are called meridians. Unfortunately, these meridians are not maintenance-free. Things like a bad diet, stress, or viruses can obstruct them. When that happens, your energy flow becomes unbalanced, which results in injury or disease. To regain balance, Chinese medicine teaches that you have to stimulate special points along the meridians, known as acupoints, which enhance or alter the flow of qi and restore balance and health.

What to Expect

Like any doctor, an acupuncturist will take your history upon your first visit, though the questions are a bit different from what you might expect. You will be asked about your urine color, menstrual cycle, sensitivity to temperature and the seasons, eating and sleeping habits, digestive problems, and even your emotional state. The practitioner will check the color of your skin and hair, will observe the coating on your tongue, and will also note your tone of voice, body language, body odor, and any other signs of imbalance. He or she will also take an extended reading of your pulse, Chinese-medicine style, checking twelve points along your wrist.

After analyzing the information gathered during this broad history, the practitioner will make a diagnosis and then proceed with the treatment. Though people unfamiliar with acupuncture tend to expect the process to be painful, much like receiving a shot with a hypodermic needle, the acupuncture needling process is actually quite painless. The needles themselves are extremely thin and flexible. Most people report nothing more than a slight pricking when the needle is inserted, and then they feel only minor tightness or heaviness around the point of insertion once the needle is in place, rather than pain.

During a typical treatment, you will lie down on a table while several needles are inserted at the appropriate acupoints. After about twenty minutes the practitioner will remove the needles. Many people report feeling a sense of relaxation bordering on euphoria following treatment. How many treatment sessions you will need will depend upon the condition. As a rule, acute problems like pain from an injury will require only a few sessions, while chronic problems like allergies will require a longer treatment regimen.

When East Meets West

Of course, if you start talking to Western doctors about your qi being blocked, they're likely to give you a dose of Maalox and tell you to take a long weekend to recover. Being more clinically analytical, most doctors want to know why and how acupuncture "really" works before they will believe.

Though Western medicine hasn't universally accepted acupuncture, some research is providing answers. Clinical studies have shown that acupuncture reduces pain by triggering the release of natural opiate-like painkillers in the body known as endorphins and enkephalins. It can also help release other chemicals such as adrenocorticotropic hormone (ACTH), which helps fight inflammation; prostaglandins, which may help to heal wounds more quickly; and various other substances that help the body to regenerate nerves.

Although such findings explain how acupuncture can act as an anesthetic against pain, how it treats other conditions is still largely a mystery. Despite some unanswered questions, plenty of American medical doctors have put faith in this ancient Chinese secret. A full one-third of the 9,000 practicing acupuncturists in this country have the title M.D.

One of the biggest nods of approval for acupuncture has been given by the government—namely the United States Food and Drug Administration (FDA). After reviewing the data on this ancient mode of healing, the FDA reclassified acupuncture needles from "investigational," meaning that they still require clinical study for approval, to "general use for licensed, registered, or certified acupuncture practitioners." This means that acupuncture needles have joined the ranks of scalpels and syringes as legitimate medical equipment.

Although the FDA has not officially acknowledged that acupuncture is an effective treatment for any specific ailment, that day may not be far off. Currently, only about three dozen of the 2,500 published studies on acupuncture meet Western standards, but clinical studies are underway that are making a case for using acupuncture to treat conditions of all kinds, from migraines and asthma to arthritis and addiction.

What It Treats

The American Association of Acupuncture and Oriental Medicine (AAAOM) documents more than forty conditions commonly treated with acupuncture, though only a few have been confirmed by results from Western medical studies. Acupuncturists generally say that acupuncture is most effective for managing chronic diseases, such as low back pain and asthma. Here are a few of the areas where acupuncture is considered most effective.

Asthma—Because it is effective in easing inflammation, acupuncture can be useful for controlling asthma, which involves inflammation of the lungs. After reviewing sixteen studies that tested treatments for chronic asthma and other lung diseases, researchers concluded that acupuncture is a safe and potentially effective treatment. Ten of the studies found that acupuncture could help people who have asthma significantly reduce their need for medication.

Chronic pain—From migraines to backaches, the best-documented benefits of acupuncture are in the area of pain management. In one major study, acupuncture provided short-term relief for 55 to 85 percent of people who were suffering from chronic pain.

Migraine headaches have been the focus of much acupuncture research. In one typical experiment some Austrian researchers found that out of twenty-six migraine sufferers, eighteen reported fewer bouts with headache following acupuncture and fifteen still felt headache relief three years later.

ACUPUNCTURE ALERT

Before you visit an acupuncturist, here are some things to consider.

See your doctor. If you have a serious illness, always see your physician before seeking alternative care. While your doctor will likely give you the go-ahead to seek acupuncture, some conditions such as acute infections, cancer, and heart disease cannot be treated by needles alone.

Know your needles. Your acupuncturist should use standard disposable needles that are individually packaged in plastic. The needles should not be opened until the practitioner is ready to insert them in your skin.

Check credentials. Most of the best practitioners, whether Eastern or Western, are found through referrals. Check for a reputable acupuncturist from one of the organizations listed earlier.

Be prepared to pay. Although the tide is slowly turning, the majority of states still do not mandate that insurance companies cover acupuncture treatments. So be prepared to pick up the tab. Your first visit to an acupuncturist can cost anywhere from forty up to one hundred dollars.

Stick with it. Stay realistic in your expectations. Even if acupuncture is successful for you, chances are one treatment won't do the trick. Give it a try for five to ten treatments. If after that point you're not feeling better, opt for another acupuncturist or try another type of healing.

Stick with your doctor, too. If the acupuncturist advises you to stop seeing your doctor or stop taking your medication, head for the exit. Medicine should be a complementary process.

Acupuncture also is frequently used in the treatment of pain caused by fibromyalgia (musculoskeletal pain), arthritis, sports injuries, disk problems, toothache, tendinitis, bursitis, and angina. It has even been used successfully to facilitate life support before surgery as well as to provide post-operative pain relief.

Menopause and menstrual problems—Though more research is needed, one small study of twenty-one menopausal women found that acupuncture treatment cut the number of hot flashes these women experienced by more than half. Other studies have found that women suffering from dysmenorrhea—pain during menstruation—can often get relief through acupuncture.

Substance abuse—One place where acupuncture has made major inroads on the path to mainstream medical acceptance is in the treatment of drug addiction. Experts believe that it's acupuncture's endorphin-producing ability that makes it such an effective addiction fighter. By stimulating the brain's natural calming agents, needle treatments lessen the need for a "fix." Some of the clearest evidence of acupuncture's power over addiction comes from a study involving two groups of forty people suffering from alcohol addiction. One group received real acupuncture treatments, while the other group received placebo or "sham" treatments, or acupuncture needles placed in the wrong locations. Remarkably, twenty-one of the forty people who received the real treatments finished the eight-week program, while only one of those receiving bogus treatments hung on till the end. And six months later, the people from the acupuncture group reported just half as many drinking episodes as those from the placebo treatment group.

Based on those kinds of results, one of the first treatment recommendations offenders are given in drug courts is to receive acupuncture. According to the National Acupuncture Detoxification Association in Washington, D.C., there are nearly 2,500 acupuncture addiction specialists spread across the country. In New York alone, more than ninety treatment programs include acupuncture.

Future Uses

Acupuncture's potential for healing is truly great. Conditions ranging from hypertension to diabetes to depression may all be relieved by the pricking of an acupuncturist's needle. As the public enthusiasm for this ancient method grows, more research dollars will be available to forge new insights into how acupuncture works and where it works best.

ACUPRESSURE: RELIEF AT YOUR FINGERTIPS

If you have ever rubbed your temples to relieve a pounding headache, you may understand the reasoning behind acupressure—a technique practiced in the Far East even before the advent of acupuncture needles. But despite its antiquity, acupressure is still considered a powerful healer.

Acupressure uses the same meridian/acupoint philosophy as acupuncture does, but with a twist: Because it does not involve needles it can be used as a simple home remedy, experts say. If your ankle is injured, for instance, you can apply gentle acupressure around the swollen joint to open up channels and increase circulation in that area. Like acupuncture, when done correctly acupressure is not very painful; it's supposed to feel like a "good hurt."

What It Treats

Nausea—Aside from treating injuries, acupressure has been clinically proven to control nausea. Pregnant women, people undergoing surgery, and folks prone to motion sickness can all benefit from using acupressure to calm their stomachs.

In one study of sixty pregnant women, researchers found that pressure applied to a spot on the wrist, called the *Nei Guan* point, significantly reduced morning sickness. One-half of the women in the study were told to press on the

Nei Guan point four times a day for seven days, while the other women were instructed to apply pressure to a bogus point, where no known meridians or acupoints exist. At the study's end, the women applying acupressure to an actual Nei Guan point were much less nauseated, while the women applying pressure to the phony point still felt sick. As a result, many major medical centers now recommend that their patients who are troubled by morning sickness try Sea-Bands or AcuBands—wristbands sold in nautical and some natural health stores—which prevent nausea by applying pressure to the Nei Guan point.

These bands also can be effective in fighting nausea from causes other than morning sickness, such as the queasiness people commonly feel after surgery. One study of forty-one people undergoing laparoscopic surgery had nineteen wear AcuBand pressure straps on their wrists, while the other twenty-one wore fake bands. Among those wearing the fake bands, ten patients felt sick and six vomited. Among those wearing the real bands, only six felt nauseated and none vomited. You might also want to try these bands for long car rides, since they are also effective against motion sickness.

Pain and tension—Acupressure has been successful in relieving all kinds of headaches, fatigue, stress, and menstrual and menopausal discomforts. Some health and beauty spas offer facial acupressure to relieve tension in your face and improve circulation under the skin to make your face glow.

FOR MORE INFORMATION

As with most health care methods, there are different regulations for different states. Look for someone with either two years of training at an accredited school, at least four years of experience as an apprentice, or an M.D. who has a minimum of 200 hours of training. The following organizations can help you.

The Acupressure Institute
1533 Shattuck Avenue
Berkeley, California
800-442-2232

American Association of Oriental Medicine
(AAOM)
433 Front Street
Catasauqua, Pennsylvania 18032
610-266-1433

American Academy of Medical Acupuncture
(AAMA)
5820 Wilshire Blvd., Suite 500
Los Angeles, California 90036
800-521-2262

National Acupuncture and Oriental Medicine
Alliance (NAOMA)
14637 Starr Road SE
Olalla, Washington 98359
206-851-6896

National Acupuncture Detoxification Association
(NADA)
3115 Broadway, Suite 51
New York, New York 10027
(or 3220 N Street, NW, Suite #275,
Washington, D.C. 20007)

AROMATHERAPY

The Scent of Good Health

If you have ever walked into a bakery and were instantly transported to the warm, cozy security of your grandmother's house, you understand the basic idea of aromatherapy: Smell, or aroma, has the power to make us feel better.

Though it is often categorized as a "new age" remedy, aromatherapy—the use of essential oils from aromatic plants for healing—dates back thousands and thousands of years. Jesus made reference to aromatic oils in the Bible. King Tut and Queen Nefertiti were firm believers in the benefits of rose baths and oils. European healers in the eleventh century used oils to help prevent and cure disease. And countless spiritual ceremonies, from weddings and baptisms to funerals, have been and are still blessed with essential oils.

Given the long, rich history of aromatherapy, it should be no surprise that researchers in Japan have found that the fragrances from many natural oils can actually change your brain waves to make you feel more alert and focused in some cases and more calm and relaxed in others. Likewise, English researchers have found that the scent of lavender can lift the spirits of patients in an intensive care unit. Even our own stodgy corporate culture is following its nose to the potential benefits of aromatherapy. Some companies pipe relaxing, fragrant blends into their office lobbies to soothe the nerves of frazzled visitors. And that's merely scratching the surface of what the right scents can do for your well-being.

The Nose Knows

The olfactory nerve—found in the upper regions of the nasal cavity—provides the most direct route to your limbic system, the brain's emotional mainframe and the warehouse of stored memories. That's why one whiff from a bakery, a pine forest, or a familiar perfume can open your emotional floodgates, allowing poignant mental reminders to come rushing into your mind. The limbic system is also directly connected to those parts of the brain that control heart rate, blood pressure, breathing, stress levels, and hormone balance. It's not hard to believe that one of the most effective ways to manipulate these metabolic functions is right under your nose.

And, when you inhale a fragrance from a natural oil, particles from the substance are absorbed directly through the linings of the nose and the lungs into your bloodstream. If applied topically, particles from some essential oils can act like a cleanup crew, killing harmful bacteria. Other essential oils can recharge your brain cells. Scientists can actually measure the different parts of the brain that each scent affects. Orange, jasmine, and rose, for instance, alter brain waves in a way that calms you down and increases your sense of well-being, while oils like rosemary and black pepper are more stimulating and increase your energy.

Interestingly, though a host of fragrances, natural and artificial, may be pleasing to your nose, only natural essences actually alter brain waves, Japanese researchers have found. Though that floral air freshener may make your home smell nice, it won't give you the benefits of aromatherapy.

Not Just for Smelling

Like many medicines, essences can be used in a variety of ways. They can be particularly effective when you rub them on your skin. As you might expect, when used topically, oils can treat a wide array of skin problems. Their astringent, antiseptic properties make them good for killing infectious germs on cuts and abrasions. They can also nourish aging,

11

dry, or cracked skin. Because they're made of tiny molecules, they actually penetrate the skin and enter your bloodstream, providing healing effects inside as well as outside.

Scents for Good Health

Once you start investigating aromatherapy you will find a forest full of scents. There's no need to be overwhelmed. You can reap substantial benefits from aromatherapy by choosing just a few select oils. The following primer will help you understand the most commonly used essences and what they are good for.

Basil—Derived from the leaves and flowering plant tops, basil is uplifting and refreshing. Using basil in the bath is popular in Ayurvedic medicine (an Ancient Indian philosophy enjoying renewed popularity) for cooling and warming the skin simultaneously. Some folks also recommend it as an insect repellent.

Black pepper—A stimulating essence, black pepper is good for increasing energy. It's derived from the unripe fruit and berry of peppercorn.

Cedar wood—Like the scent of hope chests, cedar wood is a sweet fragrance that clears the mind. Topically, it is good for relieving itchy skin, as well as working as an astringent and antiseptic.

Citrus oils—Having a party? Diffuse some citrus essence into the air. Aromatherapists recommend cheerful citrus oils for chasing away foul moods and creating a bright, uplifting atmosphere. Citrus oils are also fairly inexpensive. Grapefruit, orange, lemon, and lime can cost as little as five dollars for five milliliters.

Clary sage—Obtained from herbs and flowers, clary sage is commonly used to combat depression, menstrual pain, and premenstrual syndrome. When diffused into the air or used as a massage oil, this essence is said to make you euphoric.

Eucalyptus—Remember that soothing rub your mother applied to your chest when you were sick as a child? It was the eucalyptus oil in it that helped clear your congestion. Eucalyptus is a classic antiviral and expectorant used in aromatherapy treatments.

Floral oils—Hands down, floral oils are the best for stress relief, say aromatherapists. You can buy floral oils in just about any price range, from the rare and expensive rose oil to the more common and affordable geranium oil.

Geranium—This floral essence is not only relaxing and inexpensive, but it has special properties as an antiviral and antifungal agent. It also tends to be gentle on the skin, so it works well for topical treatments.

Lavender—If you could buy only one essential oil, aromatherapy experts agree it should be lavender. Studies in hospital intensive care units show that this fragrant oil can improve mood and relieve stress. Plus, lavender is an excellent first-aid oil. Apply it undiluted to minor injuries like small burns, cuts, bruises, and insect bites. Because it contains the sedative compound ester, some people put a drop or two on their bedsheets to relieve minor insomnia.

Mandarin—One of the most popular citrus oils, mandarin oil is a top choice to ease anxiety and raise your spirits.

Niaouli—This essential oil calms respiratory allergies. It is vitalizing, and when used topically it can provide relief for oily skin. Some people also find it works well on minor hemorrhoid problems.

Palmarosa—Sometimes used topically in the treatment of herpes, palmarosa oil has excellent antiseptic and antiviral uses, and is a staple in many aromatherapy mixtures.

Patchouli—This spicy smelling essential oil is used to calm and focus the mind. Patchouli also soothes dry skin and some people find it has an aphrodisiac quality.

Peppermint—Peppermint is one of the essential oils that

AROMATHERAPY ALERT

Though generally safe, most aromatherapy oils are still medicinal and can cause side effects, especially if you're using them directly on your skin. Typical problems include allergic reaction or irritation due to excessive use of oils that can potentially trigger allergies, such as clove, cinnamon, oregano, and savory. The following tips will help you enjoy aromatherapy without such side effects.

Smell, don't taste. Some oils can have medicinal benefits if taken internally, but others like hyssop, sage, and mugwort can be toxic. Your best bet is to use them on your own only as fragrances. See a professional aromatherapist if you're interested in learning more about how to use them internally.

Take a pregnant pause. Pregnant women should consult with their doctors before using any kind of aromatherapy. Calamus, mugwort, pennyroyal, sage, and wintergreen can induce miscarriage when taken internally. Doctors caution against using these oils in any form if you're pregnant. Other essences that should be avoided during pregnancy are basil, hyssop, myrrh, marjoram, and thyme.

Conduct a test. You should always conduct a skin patch test before applying essential oils to your skin, because some of them can cause irritation or allergic reactions in sensitive people—particularly people with fair or freckled skin. To perform a patch test, simply put a drop of essential oil on a cotton swab and dab it on a sensitive patch of skin, such as your inner wrist or inner elbow. Cover the patch with a bandage and don't wash it for twenty-four hours. If there is no redness or irritation at that point the oil is likely to be okay to use on your skin.

works well when it is taken internally—though you should consult an expert before trying it yourself. A drop on the tongue provides relief from nausea and travel sickness. Topically, it cools and invigorates the skin. Breathing in the vapors from two or three drops of peppermint essence in a bowl of hot water can provide relief from colds, flu, or sinus congestion. Finally, it is a great mental stimulant.

Rose—Derived from rose petals, essential rose oil is rare and expensive. It's recommended for healing liver, stomach, and blood disorders. It's also a great stress reliever and mood elevator.

Rosemary—Used topically, rosemary oil stimulates the metabolism of the outermost layer of skin, increasing cell regeneration and improving skin quality. The fresh aroma also soothes and relieves anxiety.

Sandalwood—Obtained from the tree, sandalwood oil baths are used in aromatherapy to keep the immune system running at peak condition. Sandalwood is also an antiseptic.

Spearmint—Breathing in the vapors from this essential oil energizes the mind, and spreading it on topically cools and invigorates the skin. It's also good for toning oily skin.

Tea tree—Acting as a gentle antiseptic, tea tree oil is commonly used for skin conditions like burns, cold sores, and athlete's foot. It's added to lip balms, soaps, and dental products. Tea tree oil is also an effective antibacterial and antifungal agent.

Ylang-ylang—As one of the floral essences, ylang-ylang is excellent for soothing the body physically and mentally.

Where to Purchase Them

Aromatherapy is perfect for at-home treatment. Most health food stores carry aromatherapy oils, as do many bath and beauty specialty shops. Look for starter kits containing the most versatile and common essential oils with directions on how to use them. Essential oils vary widely in cost and quality. Most popular home-care oils are priced in the range of five to sixteen dollars for a five-milliliter bottle. Because you only use the oils a couple of drops at a time, a bottle this size typically lasts for a few months of normal use.

How to Use Them

Here are a few ways to enjoy more aromatic fragrances in your life.

Heat some water. If you live in an apartment or are interested in scenting a small room, all you need to do is add a few drops of oil to a bowl of hot water. The vapors will release the fragrance into the air.

Spray some on. For a quick burst of fragrance, take a small plant misting bottle, fill it with water, and add some essential oil. This works especially well with gentle floral oils. You can spray the air, or even use the mister to spray onto skin that is too sensitive to touch.

Use a diffuser. For around fifty dollars you can buy an aromatherapy diffuser that disperses micro-particles of the essential oil into the air. Diffusers are useful for respiratory conditions like cold, flu, and asthma, or they can simply add an uplifting energy to the air.

Take a bath. Because oils are easily absorbed through the skin, one of the nicest ways to get them in the air as well as through your skin is to add them to your steamy bath water.

Here's the rub. You can also use them in massage oils or in hot or cold compresses to soothe minor aches and pains.

For More Information

The following are some places to contact if you're looking for more information about aromatherapy or would like to find a qualified aromatherapist.

The Pacific Institute of Aromatherapy
P.O. Box 6842
San Rafael, California 94903
415-479-9121

National Association for Holistic Aromatherapy
P.O. Box 17622
Boulder, Colorado 80308-0622

Lotus Light
P.O. Box 1008
Silver Lake, Wisconsin 53170
414-889-8501

AYURVEDA

Healing for Your Body Type

If you've ever gone on a group vacation, you understand the old saying, "Different strokes for different folks." Some will always be cold, no matter how warm the air, while other people never stop sweating no matter how cool the breeze. Some people will pour hot sauce on every mouthful they eat, while others turn down anything spicier than mayonnaise. According to the philosophy of the ancient traditional system of medicine from India called Ayurveda, that's because different people have different biological makeups, which not only affect their food and clothing needs but also their health care needs.

The Constitution of Health

Founded in a set of spiritual texts called the Vedas, created five thousand years ago, Ayurveda (which means "the science of life") has recently been making inroads in the United States. The cornerstone of Ayurveda is the body's constitution. Practitioners of Ayurveda prescribe herbs, meditation, exercise, diet, cleansing, and many other remedies to treat their patients' specific metabolic constitutions.

"Constitution" is a little different in this sense than what you may be thinking. Ayurveda teaches that everyone is made of different combinations of the five basic elements in the universe: space, air, water, fire, and earth. These elements naturally occur in pairs called *doshas*. There are three doshas:

vata (space and air), *pitta* (fire a.
and earth). According to Ayurvec
up your mother and father combi
ments when you were conceived to
constitution, or metabolic body type.
pakruti. Though everyone's pakruti c
each dosha, most people have two dos.
with one being dominant.

While your pakruti remains constant
are born, your body is not immune to t
changing seasons and alterations in your diet
or lifestyle. These outside elements form yc
constitution, what Ayurveda refers to as your a
your vikriti should mirror your pakruti exactly.
can be thrown off balance by a number of thing
particularly poor nutrition, overwork, and other s
your environment. The result of the vikriti being un
ranges from making you feel a bit out of sorts to
making you ill.

As a rule of thumb, you're most likely to become c
balance from an excess of your dominant dosha. That
you're primarily a pitta, you're most likely to end up with
excess of pitta elements and may become sick as a result.
achieve balance, you need to determine your dominant dosh.
and adjust your diet and lifestyle in a way that counteracts or
decreases the elements present in that dosha. By living in
balance, you should achieve longevity, happiness, and good
health, according to Ayurvedic gurus.

Vata, Pitta, and Kapha

Living in balance requires understanding the three primary
doshas, how they determine your actions and reactions, and
how they are affected by practically everything in your environment. In general, it helps to relate the doshas to their
closest Western equivalents. People who are predominantly
vatas are most like "ectomorphs," or thin, light body types.

e similar to muscular, medium-build "mesomorphs." aphas are more the equivalent of softer, heavy-set norphs." But as you will discover, the doshas describe more about you than your physical body type. The ing is a descriptive guide to the doshas. (To determine primary dosha, see What's Your Dosha? on p. 24.)

The many faces of vata. Composed of space and air, s' primary characteristic is changeability. Vatas are vivaus, energetic, imaginative, and moody. Though most vatas ckly and enthusiastically grasp new tasks, follow-through another story, as vatas are quick to switch interests midream to something new. They are generally very tall or very hort, have prominent bony features, cool, dry skin, and thin hair. When thrown off balance, vatas become anxious and even fearful.

Physically, an excess of vata causes diseases associated with too much air and space, such as intestinal gas, rough skin, chapped lips, achy or arthritic joints, insomnia, and fatigue. Vatas are also the first to go out of balance and the hardest to reel back in line. Because of their tendency toward flights of fancy, vata-dominant people also have trouble adhering to a dosha-balancing diet for any length of time.

As a rule, vatas are exceedingly sensitive to the effects of sugar, alcohol, and drugs, so they should use these substances sparingly, if at all. What vatas need more than anything is grounding, which they can get from warm, cooked foods and warming spices, especially during fall and winter when vatas are most at-risk of becoming off-kilter. Because vata is the first of the doshas to go off balance, it's important for vata-dominant people to try to establish steady routines.

Type "A" pitta. Where fire meets water, you get the steam-powered, determined personality that is pitta. Embodying the characteristics of astute business people, pittas are typically intelligent, intense, orderly, and efficient. Though their extreme hunger keeps them from ever missing

a meal, pitta people don't have trouble keeping their weight down because of their energetic metabolisms. Physically, they tend to be of medium build and have fair, thin hair and warm, ruddy complexions.

When unbalanced, pittas may tend to fly off the handle, become compulsive or self-destructive, and develop conditions associated with fire and water, such as ulcers, fevers, and inflammations; and irritations like colitis, sore throats, and infections. Pittas have a tendency toward excess and often crave those very same things that throw them off balance, like spicy, hot foods, which they should clearly avoid.

Ideally, pittas should seek to cool their fiery jets, particularly in prime pitta season—summer. Their best foods are sweet, cooling fare such as mint tea, sweet fruits, and cottage cheese. They also live most happily in seasonal climates, such as the Northeast.

Slow and steady kapha. Ample, soft, and sensuous are some of the best words to describe the most down-to-earth dosha. Kapha is a combination of water and earth. Like dew-quenched soil, kapha people are cool and slow moving. Given their sweet, sleepy, relaxed nature, kaphas have a natural tendency to carry some excess weight. They also tend to have thick, wavy hair and cool, thick, oily skin.

When a kapha person becomes too kapha-heavy, however, these lovable traits can become excessive and turn "steady and slow" into "stubborn and lazy." Often, they'll seek emotional comfort through food. Too much kapha can cause conditions such as obesity, high cholesterol, sinus problems, allergies, and a tendency toward procrastination. They're also more prone to colds and flu, especially during winter, which is the primary kapha season.

To maintain balance, kaphas should strive to eat plenty of bitter or astringent foods, resisting their natural urge to indulge in fatty, sweet, or oily victuals. Kaphas thrive best in warm environs such as the desert plains of the Southwest.

What to Expect

A visit to an Ayurvedic practitioner bears little resemblance to a visit to a Western physician. Lab tests, blood work, and body scans using high-tech equipment are not part of the diagnostic process. Instead, practitioners spend a great deal of time observing and examining the body visually and physically. They pay special attention to the pulse, tongue, eyes, and fingernails. Interestingly, Ayurveda specialists identify three distinct types of pulse—also called vata, pitta, and kapha—and they examine six pulse points on each wrist to determine how well your internal organs are functioning.

Similarly, a practitioner will study ten points on the tongue that correspond to your internal organs. By observing the coating and color of the tongue, Ayurvedic doctors can tell if one or more of your doshas is out of balance. A white coating, for example, would indicate an excess of kapha, while brown or dark discolorations indicate a vata imbalance. Likewise, the shape, color, and condition of the fingernails are all good indications of a person's state of balance. It's also not uncommon for an Ayurvedic practitioner to feel an organ he or she believes is not functioning properly. If they suspect a problem with your liver, for instance, they might ask you to lie down on the table while pressing on the area of the organ.

Finally, you'll likely be asked to provide a sample of your first morning's urine for examination, as urine plays an important role in determining dosha imbalances. Ayurvedic practitioners believe that by using their powers of observation, they can detect imbalances that will eventually lead to disease long before the illness would ever be detected by Western medicine. Disease prevention is the foundation of Ayurveda. In fact, Ayurvedic doctors in India used to be paid only while their patients were well. If they got sick, their doctors had to cure them in order to get paid.

Regaining Your Balance

Once your imbalance has been determined, an Ayurvedic physician will help you regain your dosha balance through a series of restorative processes, which include detoxification and cleansing, palliation, rejuvenation, and also mental and spiritual healing. Included in these various processes are some recommendations for dietary changes, exercise, herbal preparations, meditation, yoga, massage, breathing exercises, and other lifestyle modifications.

Detoxification and cleansing—One of the byproducts of dosha imbalance is that it inhibits effective digestion, say Ayurvedic doctors. Over time, this can result in a buildup of toxins called *ama*—a sticky, noxious residue that gradually clogs up the cells. To detoxify the body and rid it of ama, you need to undergo what is called panchakarma in Ayurveda.

Panchakarma is an intricate purifying system that will begin with oleation therapy, or *snehana*, which involves taking large quantities of *ghee*—or clarified butter—over several days to loosen impurities. Oleation is then followed by an oil massage, called *abhyanga*, during which you are rubbed down with sesame seed oil to improve your circulation and to concentrate the toxins and excess doshas into the center of your body. Other methods for releasing toxins in your body include steam baths, known as *swedana*; shirodhara, a process of pouring warm sesame oil across your forehead in a thin, steady stream; and nasya, which is a special treatment to clear the head and neck through steam inhalation and herbal solutions dropped into the nostrils.

Once toxins are loosened and centralized and the body is calm, the toxins are then purged through a technique known as *basti*. This is a medicated enema that eliminates toxins that have been deposited in the intestinal tract. Basti is considered one of the most important components of panchakarma. Basti also is useful for balancing the vata dosha, which is often off-kilter.

WHAT'S YOUR DOSHA?

The following are the primary characteristics of the three Ayurvedic doshas: vata, pitta and kapha. To determine which is most like you, put a check by the descriptions that best suit your appearance, personality and behavior. If one column has many more checks than the others, you're likely a single-dosha type. If no one dosha clearly dominates, you are most likely a two-dosha type, with a nearly equal amount of two dosha traits and some of the third. If all three are nearly equal, you're considered to be tridoshic in Ayurveda, but this is very rare, so you may want to try once more with the input of a close friend.

VATA

Dry, curly hair; usually medium or light brown

Dry skin

Thin, bony physique

Hyperactive

Moody

Dislike cold

Imaginative

Light sleeper

Irregular appetite

Impulsive spender

Intuitive

Sensitive to noise

Anxious and fearful under stress

Tendency toward nervous disorders

PITTA	KAPHA
Straight, fine hair; blond, red, or early gray	Thick, bouncy hair; dark brown or black
Ruddy, warm complexion	Oily, smooth skin
Medium build, muscular	Heavyset build
Orderly	Slow and steady
Intense	Relaxed
Dislike heat	Dislike damp and cold Tolerate extremes well
Intelligent	Affectionate
Sound, moderate sleeper	Deep, long sleeper
Always hungry	Eat slowly
Careful with money	Save and accumulates money but will spend
Articulate	Compassionate
Sensitive to bright light	Sensitive to strong odors
Irritated under stress	Mostly calm under stress
Tendency toward ulcers, heartburn.	Tendency toward obesity.

Palliation—Employing a combination of yoga, herbs, fasting, chanting, and meditation, palliation is designed to soothe the soul and provide spiritual healing. For people too weak to undergo the physical rigors of panchakarma, palliation can be a worthwhile substitute.

Rejuvenation—Once the body is cleansed, it needs to be toned so it works optimally again. According to Ayurveda, the best way to do this is through rejuvenation treatments, which restore vitality through herbal preparations in the form of pills, jellies, powders, and tablets.

Mental and spiritual hygiene and healing—The final steps in this regimen for balance include treatments to alter the state of consciousness and release stress and negativity. These include therapies based on meditation, sound, gems, metal, and crystal therapy.

Making It Routine

To maintain perfect balance, Ayurvedic philosophy teaches that you should adhere as closely as possible to the following daily routine.

•Rise early, preferably between 5:30 and 6:30 a.m.

•Meditate every morning and afternoon for twenty minutes or more.

•Eat a mostly meatless diet, saving your main meal of the day for lunch time when your digestive fires are strongest, and sticking to a light dinner between the hours of five and six o'clock.

•Take short walks after eating to aid digestion.

•Do something enjoyable before bedtime, such as listening to music, visiting with friends, or reading.

•Go to sleep early, preferably before ten o'clock.

A Good Complement

Obviously, if you have an acute condition, Ayurveda should not be the first line of defense. But Ayurvedic doctors believe

that for some common chronic or degenerative conditions such as asthma, allergies, digestive problems, fatigue, and arthritis, they offer the perfect complement to Western medicine, which often does not handle such ailments effectively on its own.

Many of the most important components for treatment and prevention of disease are actually quite simple, yet are simultaneously the most difficult for people in our culture to do—things like going to bed early and waking up early, making time for daily meditation, eating foods that are good for you rather than those you think taste good, and avoiding harmful habits such as smoking and drinking too much. An Ayurvedic practitioner will teach you how to make these changes more easily, according to your metabolic body type.

FOR MORE INFORMATION

There are not many trained Ayurvedic practitioners in the United States, and the few to be found can only consult with clients, not technically practice medicine. If you are looking for disease treatment, you're best off consulting a medical doctor who combines Western medicine with Ayurveda. The following organizations can help.

Ayurvedic and Naturopathic Medical Clinic
2115 112th Avenue NE
Bellevue, Washington 98004
425-453-8022

Ayurvedic Institute
11311 Menaul NE, Suite A
Albuquerque, New Mexico 87112
505-291-9698

The Raj
1734 Jasmine Avenue
Fairfield, Iowa 52556
800-248-9050

BIOFEEDBACK

Your Brain over Pain

Anyone who has ever been in pain has surely tried talking themselves into feeling better. "This headache's not so bad," you think, as you rub your tender temples. "Maybe if I just relax and think happy thoughts, the pounding will go away." "Yeah, right," your more cynical self chimes in, as your head throbs on and on.

But not so fast. As far-fetched as it might seem at first glance, doctors and scientists are discovering that you can use your mind, not only to ease pain of all kinds, but also to reduce stress, control asthma, heal injuries, and even relieve symptoms of conditions like congestive heart failure, stroke, and attention deficit disorder.

The system is called biofeedback. It's a physician-guided technique that uses a modern machine, electronics, and some practice to teach you how to consciously regulate normally unconscious bodily functions—such as heart rate, breathing, and blood pressure—to control and treat a growing number of ailments, especially stress-related pain.

It is important that a skilled practitioner train the user. The idea is that after you learn how to do the process and how it should feel when done right, you will eventually be able to elicit the very same physical responses on your own without the machine.

What to Expect

This is how it works. Say you suffer from tension headaches. Using electrodes attached to your forehead, a biofeedback practitioner would wire you to a box about the size of a stereo amplifier called an electromyograph, or EMG. This device records the electrical impulses from your facial muscles and translates them into visual or auditory cues, such as a flashing lighted line or beeps of varying tones. Just as an electrocardiograph, or an EKG (another machine often used for biofeedback), allows you to "watch" and "hear" your heart as it beats, an EMG allows you to "see" and "hear" your pain, or at least the body stress that's causing it. You would then be shown how to control and manipulate the muscle tension that is causing your headache by consciously altering the blips and beeps on the screen. Once you've mastered this skill, you'll be able to control the tension without the use of the machine, say experts.

Other commonly used biofeedback monitoring devices include a skin temperature monitor (ST), which responds to blood flow beneath the skin; a galvanic skin response monitor (GSR), which reacts to the electrical conductivity of the skin; a heart rate monitor such as an EKG, which is influenced by heartbeat; and a brain wave monitor called an electroencephalogram (EEG), which responds to changes in brain wave activity.

Biofeedback is not something you should do at home initially. The brain wave machines currently are hard to find and prohibitively expensive, depending on where you live and what type and condition of machine you want to purchase. Practitioners are working, though, on making home machines more readily available, and less costly. The exceptions are blood pressure and heart rate monitors, which you can indeed buy from pharmacy stores for less than $100 and which can be used fairly easily at home.

There are as many ways to alter these unconscious body activities as there are ways to monitor them. Depending on the condition you're trying to treat, you can use meditation, relaxation, and visualization to produce the desired response, whether that be a lowered heart rate, lowered body temperature, muscle relaxation, or altered brain wave activities.

What It Treats

Biofeedback was pioneered by O. Hobart Mowrer in 1938, but it wasn't until the late '60s that biofeedback researchers in California and Kansas began attracting attention. Though it is still considered to be an "alternative" form of treatment, biofeedback therapy has made great strides in the years that it's been in practice. Clinical studies show that biofeedback is useful for a wide array of conditions, ranging from easing everyday headaches to recovering motor function following a stroke. Here are some of the most well-researched areas.

Asthma—Researchers in San Francisco report that if you teach asthma sufferers how to increase the amount of air they take in with every breath, you can give them a better sense of control over their breathing and decrease their stress about having an asthma attack. In one study of seventeen people with asthma who were treated with biofeedback, researchers found that all of them made fewer visits to the emergency room, had fewer asthma attacks, and were less reliant on medication.

Attention deficit disorder—Some scientists are experimenting with ways to replace the controversial attention deficit disorder (ADD) drug, ritalin, with biofeedback. Research suggests that people with ADD tend to have brain wave patterns concentrated in the "dreamy" theta wave range, and have few brain waves working in the beta region, which is where concentration comes from. If you could learn to control your brain waves, biofeedback experts say, you could control your ADD. To do this, electrodes are attached to your scalp so you can watch your brain waves on a computer screen. Then, you learn by playing games with your brain waves. For instance, a puzzle may be put on the screen, and by generating the right kind of brain waves, you can move the puzzle pieces into the proper places, which trains your brain waves to stay more focused. Though this kind of treatment is still in its infancy and can be costly—$50 to $125 an hour—the results are promising. People not only have shown a decrease in their ADD, but also improvements in IQ scores, grades, and test scores.

Cardiovascular conditions—If you can learn to relax and consciously control your heart rate and blood pressure, you can do your heart a world of good. That much is clear. But researchers are also finding that biofeedback training can help improve circulation and reduce the shortness of breath commonly associated with congestive heart failure. Research presented at a meeting of the American Heart Association showed that in just one twenty- to thirty-minute session, twenty-five people with congestive heart failure were able to significantly lower their vascular resistance and increase the amount of blood their hearts were able to pump per beat. In addition, their breathing slowed to healthier levels. Biofeedback has also proven useful for weaning people from their hypertension medications.

Gastrointestinal disorders—Some researchers believe that biofeedback is the single most effective treatment against gastrointestinal disorders, including fecal incontinence and a common type of constipation caused by the inability to relax the pelvic floor muscles while going to the bathroom. Likewise, by learning how to strengthen and control the pelvic floor muscles—the ones you use when you "hold" your urine—people may also find they are able to control urinary incontinence with biofeedback's help.

Headache—Headaches, particularly migraines, were one of the first ailments to be treated with biofeedback. Back in the sixties scientists discovered that at the moment a woman's headache disappeared, the skin temperature on her hands would suddenly shoot up ten degrees. Scientists then learned that people could relieve their migraines by using relaxation techniques to raise their skin temperature. Clinics have since found that people can often reduce or eliminate their migraine medications once they master biofeedback.

A recent study from the Department of Psychology at the University of South Alabama in Mobile yielded remarkable results in controlling migraine headaches in children. Thirty children with migraines were divided into three groups. One group was taught how to relax and raise the skin temperature on their hands while simultaneously given biofeedback. Another group learned the relaxation and skin temperature control techniques with no biofeedback. And the third group received no treatment. After six months, 80 percent of the biofeedback group had no symptoms, 50 percent of the relaxation-only group was symptom-free, but none of the nontreatment children were symptom-free.

Insomnia—Depending on what's behind your sleepless nights, biofeedback can be a useful tool in fighting insomnia. If sleep eludes you because your nervous system just can't seem to calm down, for instance, an expert in biofeedback can use a machine or biofeedback technique to monitor and control your muscle tension and skin temperature. This will help you learn to relax your body on your own and improve your ability to sleep. If, instead, slumber eludes you due to an emotional or mental problem, biofeedback can train you how to bring your brain waves into the area most conducive to falling into a good night's sleep.

Muscular problems—Because it teaches you how to control relaxation of muscles, biofeedback is an increasingly popular remedy for the treatment of chronic back and neck pain as well as muscular and skeletal pain caused by accidents or injury.

Scoliosis—For about the same price as a traditional body brace, parents of children experiencing scoliosis may soon be able to invest in a microchip that makes use of biofeedback techniques to allow children to help "straighten" themselves, according to researchers from Hong Kong. Preliminary data on eight children showed that the device reduced the degree of spinal deformity, or curvature, by anywhere from 35 to 72 percent. Not bad, considering that traditional braces work only in about 50 percent of scoliosis patients. The device works by connecting electrodes to the chest and down the legs. If the wearer should begin to slouch, the device beeps, reminding the wearer to straighten up. If they fail to do so, the alarm sounds again, only a little bit louder. This treatment is particularly promising for children with curvatures of 25 to 45 percent, who are typically treated with a full-body brace that "pulls" the spine into place. Because this brace is typically worn for a year or more, it contributes to muscle atrophy. It's better to let the children correct the condition themselves, say biofeedback advocates, because with biofeedback they'll not only be able to run and play more like other children while undergoing treatment, but their bodies will be stronger as a result.

On the Horizon

Biofeedback is currently allowing people to control bodily functions once believed beyond our control, such as heart rate, skin temperature, brain waves, and blood pressure. Many scientists are excited about the possibility that people could learn to control even the more unconscious bodily functions, like the production of hormones or the maintenance of immunity. Watch for biofeedback to continue pushing the envelope of mind-body medicine well into the next millennium, allowing people even greater potential to directly control their own well-being. As biofeedback techniques improve, you will likely see more mainstream practitioners who incorporate safer, noninvasive biofeedback treatments into their practices.

FOR MORE INFORMATION

To find out more about biofeedback therapy or where you can locate a qualified expert who practices biofeedback, contact one of the following organizations.

Association for Applied Psychophysiology and
Biofeedback (AAPB)
10200 W. 44th Ave, #304
Wheat Ridge, Colorado 80033-2840
303-422-8436

Center for Applied Psychophysiology
Menninger Clinic
P.O. Box 829
Topeka, Kansas 66601-0829
785-350-5402

BODYWORK

Beyond Massage

If you think about it, we have always held the power to heal ourselves right in our own hands. Massage—the systematic manipulation of muscles and joints to increase relaxation and promote healing—is ancient, dating back more than five thousand years. What we have come to call "bodywork," on the other hand, is a twentieth-century creation that uses the principles of massage as a foundation to reach a new level of healing—by integrating breathing and movement techniques, and other physiological treatments to relax, align, and stimulate the body.

Bodywork techniques generally rely on the use of pressure and friction to alter muscles and soft tissues. Many also rely on manipulating specific points or reflexes in the body that bodywork practitioners believe are the centers of energy flow, balance, and muscle tension. Though techniques vary in their approach, bodywork all strives to relieve tension, reduce stress, and minimize structural imbalances.

There are few conditions that won't respond to one form of bodywork or another. Bodywork practitioners commonly treat health problems ranging from poor posture to premenstrual syndrome (PMS). And researchers have found that these healing systems are beneficial for headache, muscle ache, anxiety, asthma attacks, and high blood pressure.

The following guide can help you find the form of bodywork that is right for you.

Typical Techniques

Alexander Technique—Frederick Alexander, a turn-of-the-century Shakespearean actor, was a pioneer advocate of proper body posture. Noticing the head-down, shoulders-slumped, question-mark-shaped pose that most individuals would strike while sitting and standing, Alexander began studying the relationship between body posture—particularly of the head, neck, and back—and emotional and physical health. He found that posture could not only affect things like vocal quality, muscle tension, and proper movement and body function, but that it also appeared to help prevent and relieve such conditions as arthritis, curvatures of the spine, gastrointestinal woes, and breathing disorders. Alexander created a system of retraining and realigning the body, which was formalized in the 1970s as the Alexander Technique.

The best way to learn the Alexander Technique is with a trained instructor. Typically, the teacher will ask you to either stand, sit, or lie down while he or she helps you reposition your head, neck, and torso. You then learn specific exercises to help you maintain your newly acquired posture. After a series of lessons, students will emerge from classes with a renewed body image, improved body positioning, and, very often, better health.

BODYWORK ALERT

As healing as the various forms of bodywork can be, they are not appropriate for everyone or every condition. Always get clearance from your regular doctor before starting a new therapy.

Aston-Patterning—Stressing fitness, Aston-Patterning was developed as a follow-up therapy to help people hold onto the benefits of Rolfing. (Rolfing is discussed later in this section.) Its creator is Judith Aston, a dance instructor who used Rolfing techniques to rehabilitate herself following injuries from back-to-back motor vehicle accidents. After several years of practicing Rolfing, in the 1970s Aston developed her own system of stretching, strengthening, and realigning the body.

One of the unique elements of Aston-Patterning is its focus on the asymmetry, rather than the balance, of the body. According to Aston, everyday motions and actions require that our muscles develop in asymmetrical—or uneven—ways. Writing, playing tennis, and even driving are examples of common activities that require an unbalanced use of our muscles. Aston-Patterning practitioners focus on defining which imbalances are healthy and which may cause problems. They then use movement instruction, massage, fitness training, and environmental design—such as adjusting the height and positioning of tables and chairs to best suit different body types—to help people use their bodies in the most efficient and healthful ways.

Aston-Patterning is popular for improving movement, posture, and coordination, as well as for managing pain from injury, backaches, and headaches.

Feldenkrais—Unlike many other bodywork techniques, Feldenkrais doesn't impose its own notion of proper posture upon its participants. It accepts that people have their own posture and movement patterns, often based on self-image. Feldenkrais practitioners don't view all movement and posture as good, however. They certainly recognize that people often develop negative ways of moving and positioning their bodies. But rather than manipulating you into a "proper" position, they teach you slow, gentle exercises that naturally interrupt your old patterns of movement and replace them with new, better patterns that are more fluid. Practitioners also employ gentle massage to increase your ability to move your body through its full range of motion.

Developed by physicist Moshe Feldenkrais to heal himself from a sports-related injury, the Feldenkrais method is used today to help people rehabilitate from a wide array of conditions. These can include loss of movement from stroke, injury from motor vehicle accidents or exercise, the debilitating effects of stress, and the discomfort of back pain.

Hellerwork—Another technique designed to realign the body, this offshoot of Rolfing (see p. 40) was created by Joseph Heller, who was the first president of the Rolf Institute, to improve body movement and flexibility.

Like Rolfing, Hellerwork relies on physical manipulation by the practitioner to mend structural misalignments and improve mobility. But Hellerwork takes body realignment a few steps farther, adding an educational and mental awareness element to help make the changes stick. Heller designed an eleven-step program that begins with breathing instruction and works its way through techniques for sitting, standing, running, and generally moving in ways that work with the natural design of your body. The end result should be that you can move with minimal stress and use your energy most efficiently.

Hellerwork is useful for people who are recovering from an injury or who have pain and discomfort from stress or sore, stiff muscles.

Polarity—Polarity is known as an energy-based system. Its goal is to use massage to balance the flow of energy throughout the body. Developed by American chiropractor, naturopath, and osteopath Randolph Stone, polarity therapy was designed to harmonize the body's energy flow and structural balance by using gentle and deep manipulation. When energy is can flow freely throughout the body, practitioners say, you stay healthy. When energy is blocked by stress or trauma, you get sick.

Polarity therapists use a variety of techniques, including manipulation of various acupressure points, breathing, massage, hydrotherapy, reflexology, stretching, and exercise, to increase your body's flow of energy and its state of balance. Polarity can help prevent or treat many conditions, and can also boost your sense of well-being.

Reflexology—Your two feet contain more than fourteen thousand nerve endings, which lead to your legs, spine, brain, and various other areas of your body. Reflexologists believe that the feet—as well as the hands—are also chock-full of points that directly affect each of your internal organs. According to reflexologists, if you manipulate the spot on your foot that corresponds to your liver, your liver will immediately relax.

Developed by an American doctor, William Fitzgerald, M.D., reflexology was intended first and foremost to promote relaxation. Eliminating tension from all parts of the body through their corresponding points on the feet enables you to fend off diseases and other problems, he said. Though the science behind reflexology is still unproven, scientific evidence of its effectiveness is growing. Studies have found that it can be particularly effective against PMS, as well as hypertension and anxiety. Mostly, however, reflexology is heralded as a preventive, wellness therapy.

It's also one of the bodywork systems that you can learn to do for yourself. Though it is helpful to see a trained reflexologist to "get your feet wet," you can also buy a book that maps out the feet and their corresponding body parts and start practicing right away.

Rolfing—Like the Alexander Technique, Rolfing also is a form of bodywork designed to reeducate your body about proper posture. Unlike the Alexander Technique, this ten-step process involves proper alignment of not only your head, neck, and torso but also of your pelvis, legs, and feet. The founder of Rolfing, Ida P. Rolf, Ph.D., began to investigate the healing power of realigning the body after an alternative health practitioner cured her chronic respiratory problem by repositioning a rib that had been misaligned when she was kicked by a horse. It wasn't just trauma or injury that could cause structural misalignment, said Rolf. Repetitive movements and aging can lead to shortening of your muscles and connective tissues, as well as the resulting structural imbalance. Rolfing—the technique she developed in the 1940s—uses deep-tissue massage and manipulation of the myofacial tissue (the white connective tissue that encases muscle and connects it to your bone) along with education to improve posture and structural integrity.

Poor posture, chronic pain, structural disorders such as one shoulder sitting higher than the other, and also various curvatures of the spine, such as lordosis, are conditions that practitioners say benefit the most from Rolfing treatments.

This head-to-toe therapy is very hands-on. Rolfers use their knuckles, fingers, and elbows to stretch and lengthen your connective tissues. In the earlier days of Rolfing, this technique earned a reputation for being somewhat painful. Today, Rolfing is more tolerable as Rolfers work to use more gentle, yet equally effective manipulation.

Therapeutic touch—This is one bodywork therapy that often involves little hands-on treatment. Odd though it may seem, therapeutic touch is strictly an energy-based manipulation therapy. A combination of healing techniques such as visualization, laying on of hands, and aura therapy, therapeutic touch was developed by Dolores Krieger, Ph.D., R.N., to discharge negative energy, decrease anxiety, and reduce pain.

Typically, a therapeutic touch practitioner will hold his or her hands about two to six inches away and slowly and rhythmically work around your body, determining where you may have energy blockages. Then, the practitioner works to replenish and properly redirect the energy so your body can heal itself.

Studies indicate that therapeutic touch is very effective against headache pain. It is also frequently used to calm crying babies and to reduce women's anxiety and discomfort during their pregnancies.

Trager work—Probably the most gentle of the hands-on manipulation therapies, Trager work was developed in the 1920s by Milton Trager, M.D., as a nonintrusive way to ease neuromuscular disorders such as sciatica and even symptoms of multiple sclerosis.

Trager work simply involves lying back and allowing the Trager practitioner to work through your muscles and joints. Generally, therapists begin with your head and gradually work their way down your body, gently cradling each limb and slowly rocking and swaying the joint through its entire range of motion. Simultaneously, they massage the connecting muscles with their fingertips. To help you maintain the effects of Trager work therapy, a practitioner will also teach you Menastics, or "mental gymnastics." Menastics are slow, rhythmic, dance-like movements that are performed not by exerting your muscles, but by shifting the weight of your body and releasing the tension in your joints.

Like most bodywork therapies, Trager work is beneficial for treating a wide variety of conditions. But it is most helpful for disorders related to muscular and psychological stress.

What to Expect

Going to see a bodywork therapist is much like taking a trip to any other alternative medicine practitioner. Upon the first visit, you'll be asked to describe your reason for the visit, your medical history, your stress levels, your work conditions, your activity levels, and anything else that affects your mental and physical well-being.

The cost of treatment can range from about thirty-five to sixty dollars for an hour-long session, depending upon the type of treatment, the experience of the practitioner, and where you live. Expect to pay considerably more if you want the practitioner to make house calls.

FOR MORE INFORMATION

The following organizations can help you find a qualified bodywork therapist in your area.

American Massage Therapy Association
820 Davis Street, Suite 100
Evanston, Illinois 60201-4464
847-864-0123

National Certification Board for Therapeutic
Massage and Bodywork
P.O. Box 1080
Evanston, Illinois 60204-1080
847-864-0774

CHIROPRACTIC

Healthy Adjustments

"Oh, my aching back!" is uttered so frequently it has become a cliché. But there's good reason for this common refrain. Back pain affects more than three-quarters of us during our lifetimes. In fact, it's second only to the common cold as a reason to head to the doctor's office, and is surpassed only by childbirth as a reason to be in the hospital.

Little wonder that, despite the cloud of controversy that has historically accompanied chiropractic care, the nation's 50,000 chiropractors now compose the third-largest group of health care practitioners, outnumbered only by physicians and dentists.

But even with its prevalence and popularity, few people truly understand the fundamentals of chiropractic care or its potential for healing. In fact, chiropractors themselves even disagree on this subject. Here's what you need to know about the history and philosophy of this varied healing modality.

The Backbone of Chiropractic Care

Spinal health is the cornerstone of chiropractic care. Every civilization from the Egyptians on has practiced some form of spinal adjustment for healing. The oldest, and the most traditional school of chiropractic teaches that most diseases are caused by an out-of-place bone along the spine—known as a subluxation. This belief was touted by Daniel David Palmer, the chiropractic pioneer who founded the current system in 1895. Palmer, expert in anatomy and physiology, found he could heal a man who had been deaf for seventeen years by administering a chiropractic thrust to a misaligned vertebra. Palmer believed that people possess "innate intelligence," and that the charge of chiropractic was to alleviate nerve interference caused by subluxations, allowing a person's innate intelligence to continue its job of regulating health. He contended that because the spine is the mainframe for the network of nerves that makes up our nervous system, such spinal misalignments cause network disruptions that eventually can lead to imbalances and disease.

For example, not only can a subluxation cause physical discomfort such as muscle spasms, headaches, and muscular stress and tension, but it may interfere with the flow of nerve impulses to other parts of the body. It can prevent the liver, kidneys, or other body organs from doing their jobs properly. Though most chiropractors today don't believe that these subluxations are truly the root of all disease, there's still a large constituency—generally known in chiropractic care as "straights"—who contend that without proper spinal alignment optimal health is unachievable because the nervous system won't function at its maximum capacity. And though they don't blame misalignment for causing all disease, they hold that it is a major contributor to most.

It is here that the profession divides. There is another camp of chiropractors, known as "mixers," who mainly use the powers of chiropractic to heal the most obvious ailments related to spinal misalignment, such as back pain, neck pain, pain from trauma or injuries, and occasionally headaches. Chiropractors in this group are more likely to incorporate other natural therapies, such as massage, exercise, and nutrition, into their healing regimen.

The majority of chiropractors fall somewhere between these two ends of the spectrum. They're likely to use X-rays to detect "kinks" in the spinal column and in certain cases will recommend chiropractic care to treat problems beyond back pain. Chiropractors are not licensed to prescribe medications and cannot perform surgery. All chiropractors use spinal manipulation as their primary healing tool.

CHIROPRACTIC ALERT

Improperly applied, chiropractic treatment can be just as harmful as taking the wrong prescription drugs. Chiropractors receive careful instruction during their training on conditions that respond unfavorably to manipulation.

You should not see a chiropractor if you have any of the following conditions:
- Infection
- Inflammation
- Joint instability
- Malignant disease of the vertebrae

Chiropractic care is considered controversial for the treatment of these ailments:
- Asthma
- Dysmenorrhea
- Hypertension
- Irritable bowel syndrome

Finally, be aware that manipulation of the neck can be risky if you are taking oral contraceptives or blood-thinning medications, have high blood pressure, or are in a high-risk category for stroke.

What It Treats

The answer to the question of what chiropractic can treat largely depends upon which chiropractor you ask, because there are almost as many philosophies of the modality as there are people who practice it. There are two conditions chiropractors are most commonly called on to treat.

Addiction—One intriguing use of chiropractic is in the treatment of addiction. So far, studies have shown that people who receive chiropractic care are much more likely to complete their drug rehabilitation programs than those who don't receive chiropractic care. Though no one can say for certain how chiropractic manipulation treats addiction, many of those in the profession say that the answer lies in the nervous system. By straightening the spinal cord and removing any blockages in the nervous system pathways, this treatment gives drug-dependent people a better chance of normal nervous system functioning—without dependence on artificial substances. Some organizations that treat addiction also favor chiropractic care because it is a drug-free approach to healing.

Back pain—If you are a back pain sufferer, you may be in luck in terms of care; of all conditions commonly treated by chiropractic, this is the area that has shown the best results in clinical studies. Back pain brings chiropractors more than half their patients. That's primarily because most traditional treatments for back pain, such as bed rest and surgery, are generally ineffective. Though chiropractic therapy certainly isn't a cure-all for backaches, it has a pretty good track record for providing relief from short-term, uncomplicated back pain. Good enough, in fact, that both the American Medical Association and major medical insurers now accept chiropractic treatment as a viable therapy for back pain.

One two-year study conducted by Britain's Medical Research Council found chiropractic treatment to be more effective—both immediately and years later—than hospital outpatient care for pain in the lower back. A highly prestigious center for research in public policy, called the Rand Corporation in Los Angeles, found that spinal manipulation is indeed helpful for certain back pain sufferers.

People who are most likely to benefit from chiropractic care are those who have been in pain for less than three weeks and who have no damage to the spinal nerves leading to the legs. In these cases, spinal manipulation had people feeling better and back on their feet again more quickly than most traditional therapies. Finally, the Ontario Ministry of Health compared treatment modalities for low back pain and pronounced chiropractic manipulation to be safer, more effective, and more cost-saving than traditional medical management.

What to Expect

Like most medical practitioners, chiropractors rely on a wide array of techniques and procedures to perform diagnoses and treatments. There are almost a hundred manipulative chiropractic techniques, each with a different effect on the spine. In most cases, after taking a history of your family and personal habits, such as diet and exercise, the doctor will give a physical exam. Chiropractors generally use a combination of touch or palpation, active motion by the patient, and passive motion (with the doctor assisting the patient's movements) to make their adjustments.

One very common technique is a maneuver that involves gently stretching a joint to a point just beyond its normal range, where it gives off a painless "popping" sound caused by the release of gases from the joint fluid. Following this procedure, people generally report feeling a wider range of motion in the joint and relief from any soreness they were experiencing.

Some chiropractors prefer using subtler force. Instead of cracking and popping the vertebral subluxations, they simply apply gentle pressure along the spine, skull, and pelvis. Still others adjust not only the vertebrae but also the muscles that hold them in place.

Finding the Right Chiropractic Care

If you decide that chiropractic care is just what the doctor ordered for your aching back, then you want to be sure that you're in good hands. Experts offer the following advice for finding the right chiropractic care.

Seek someone who has "felt your pain." With so many styles, techniques, and chiropractic philosophies to choose from, you're best off finding someone who has sought chiropractic care for a condition similar to your own and asking for a referral, say experts in the field.

Work with your doctor. Although you don't need to get a physician's clearance to see a chiropractor for most simple low back pain, your chiropractor should be willing to refer you to a physician if necessary. More importantly, if it's your first time visiting a chiropractor, get a physician's evaluation first, because anything from muscle sprain to cancer can be the culprit behind an aching back. Like many other alternative therapies, chiropractic should complement, not replace, traditional medicine.

Be realistic, but set limits. Studies show that for most problems, five to ten sessions are enough to provide relief. Although you should certainly feel free to return to your chiropractor for adjustments if such treatments make you feel better, you wouldn't want to see your chiropractor fifty times a year for general health, say experts. If you are in chronic pain and the treatments don't seem to be working, you should see your regular doctor.

Get a referral. There's no need to approach chiropractic care blindly. Either get a referral from your doctor or call one of the many organizations that maintains referral lists of professionals in the field. When you have found a professional in your area, you can call ahead and make sure his or her treatment philosophy matches your own.

FOR MORE INFORMATION

Looking for a good certified chiropractor close to home? Or would you like to learn more about the profession? The following organizations can help.

American Chiropractic Association (ACA)
1701 Clarendon Boulevard
Arlington, Virginia 22209
1-800-986-4636

World Chiropractic Alliance (WCA)
2950 N. Dubson Road, Suite 1
Chandler, Arizona 85224
1-800-347-1011

DIET THERAPY

Let Food Be Thy Medicine

Folklore abounds about the medicinal properties of food. We've all heard praises sung of apples to keep us healthy, carrots to sharpen our vision, and chicken soup to soothe our winter woes. Today, you can add to these broccoli to fight cancer, soybeans to ease menopause problems, onions to prevent heart disease, and dozens more. Scientists are finally discovering the truth behind the famous advice, "Let food be thy medicine and medicine be thy food," uttered by the famous Greek physician Hippocrates more than two thousand years ago. He was truly ahead of his time.

Until recently, few of us were heeding the tried-and-true advice from generations of moms and grandmothers to eat our fruits and veggies. And we've paid the price with poor health. Statistics show that four of the ten leading causes of death in the United States—heart disease, cancer, stroke, and diabetes—are connected to what we eat. And to what we don't eat.

That's where diet therapy comes in. A growing number of doctors, nurses, dieticians, and other health care practitioners, alternative as well as mainstream, are devoting time to teaching people how to adjust their diets to fend off health foes ranging from asthma and cataracts to cancer.

Changing Diets

You'd never believe it now, but cancer used to be a rarity. Heart attack? No such thing was even documented until the beginning of the twentieth century. Before then, hardening of the arteries was so uncommon that medical textbooks did not even include it as an entry. It's no coincidence that this was also before the Industrial Revolution, when people grew what they ate and animal foods were saved for special occasions rather than being placed front and center at every meal.

Diet therapy experts agree that one of the steepest prices of progress has been what appears on our dinner plates every evening. With the spread of combustion engines and power tractors, steamboats and locomotives, farmers could grow more food, raise more livestock, and ship more food to more places around the country. Suddenly, ears of corn became corn chips, whole wheat became white bread and, decades later, processed foods became the perfect easy fare for an evening in front of the tube with Ozzie and Harriet.

When it comes to diet, people are starting to recognize that new is not necessarily better. In fact, the United States Department of Agriculture Food Pyramid, which is a model for healthy eating, remarkably resembles the way we used to eat in simpler times, before cars, television, steam engines, and heart disease. The Pyramid recommends that we eat six to eleven servings of whole-grain foods, two to three servings of fruits, and three to five servings of vegetables a day.

Fiber Up

If you had to name the thing people are missing most in these ready-to-eat, fast-food days, it would be fiber. What your grandparents used to call "roughage," doctors are now calling protection from ailments and diseases ranging from constipation to cancer.

Fiber is like your body's internal cleaning system. You don't digest it. Rather, it moves its way through your digestive tract, sweeping up the toxins, absorbing cholesterol, and adding bulk to your stools so everything your body doesn't need or want gets passed out of your system in an efficient manner. Unfortunately, the average daily dietary fiber intake in Western countries has plummeted during the past century, from forty grams 100 years ago to fifteen or twenty grams today. To reap the benefits of a fiber-filled diet, food therapy experts say, we should be aiming for more than thirty-five grams a day. The following are just a few of the conditions you can prevent or treat if you increase your fiber intake.

Colon disease and colon cancer—Getting enough roughage can protect you from a host of common digestive tract ailments. One such condition is diverticulosis, in which small pouches form in the colon that sometimes become inflamed and painful. More than one-third of all people over age forty-five have them. The good news is that in a study of 47,888 male doctors, researchers found that men who ate an average of thirty-two grams of fiber a day had nearly one-half the risk of diverticulosis as men who ate thirteen grams of fiber a day.

Swedish researchers studied eighty-two people, half with colorectal cancer and half who were cancer-free. They found that people who included the most cereal fiber in their diets had an 88 percent lower risk for colon cancer than those who ate the least.

Constipation—Fiber is the most natural kind of relief for constipation you can find. Scientists have reported that when people who normally ate low amounts of fiber added twenty grams of fiber to their diets, they increased the bulk of their stools by 127 percent and cut the time that waste stayed in the body by 41 percent. It's important, however, to be careful when adding fiber to your diet. If you up your intake all at once, you're setting yourself up for bloating and flatulence. Instead, add a few grams a day over a period of weeks, until you reach your goal.

Heart disease—Not surprisingly, with fiber's cholesterol-cutting powers, it can give heart disease a one-two punch. So much so that a group of researchers who tracked the health of a large number of men for six years found that those who ate the most fiber—about 28.9 grams a day—had approximately one-half as many heart attacks as those who ate the least fiber.

High cholesterol—Fiber binds with both dietary fat and cholesterol in the intestine, flushing them from your system before they can make their way into your bloodstream. This makes dietary fiber a perfect way to reduce cholesterol to healthy levels. In one study of thirteen volunteers with high cholesterol levels, Canadian researchers discovered that when these folks ate a breakfast cereal containing psyllium—a particularly potent type of fiber—they were able to lower their total cholesterol levels by 7.4 percent and their levels of the more dangerous low-density lipoprotein (or LDL) cholesterol by 11.1 percent in just two weeks.

DIET THERAPY ALERT

Although it never hurts to improve your eating habits, it is important to keep in mind that diet therapy is rarely a treatment in and of itself. This type of care, whether practiced at home or under the guidance of a practitioner, should be viewed as complementary to the care you receive from your regular physician.

Fat Facts

People are confused about fat. Too much fat is definitely bad. And too many people definitely eat too much. But there is bad fat and there is good fat. Eating less of the bad and more of the good will help lower your cholesterol and improve your overall health.

No one probably needs to tell you that the one fat you really should cut from your diet is saturated fat—the cholesterol-raising, artery-clogging type found in meat, cheese, and dairy products. Around the globe, researchers have found that the nations with the highest rates of breast, colon, and prostate cancer are those with the fattiest diets. Even worse, scientists have found that high-fat foods and cancer-causing toxins work together to give your body a double whammy. Animal studies have found that cancer-causing chemicals are more likely to lead to tumors in animals fed fatty foods than in those fed low-fat foods.

In an attempt to avoid high-fat dairy products, lots of people turn to alternatives, such as margarine. Unfortunately, research has found that margarine can be just as bad as saturated fat, and maybe worse. This product is made up of trans-fatty acids, or vegetable oils that have been chemically solidified so you can spread them on your toast like butter. Though it seemed like a good idea, studies have shown that your body doesn't know what to do with these foreign fats. They actually can cause a more dramatic rise in cholesterol than saturated fat.

Your best bet, then, is to stick to fats that won't be sticking to your arteries—liquid vegetable polyunsaturated and monounsaturated fats. Studies show these fats, eaten in moderation, can actually help to lower your cholesterol and help reduce inflammation. As a rule of thumb, no more than 25 percent of your calories should come from fat, with an emphasis on monounsaturated fats such as olive oil.

Health from the Garden

Hands down, the most exciting discovery diet researchers have made in the realm of food therapy pertains to fruits and vegetables. There's good news and there's better news about these oh-so-healthful foods. First, because of advances in growing, cooking, and seasoning techniques, vegetables and fruits taste better than they ever have. Second, we now know they are even better for us than we ever could have imagined.

We always knew that fruits and vegetables were chock-full of essential vitamins and minerals, but that didn't quite explain the cornucopia of health benefits these foods provided. Then researchers made a truly amazing discovery. They found that plants are armed with literally hundreds and thousands of chemicals—called phytochemicals—that protect them from bacteria, fungi, predators, and viruses. These phytochemicals not only provide benefits for the plant but also for us when we eat them. Here are some of the highlights of what they contain.

Allium sulfides—Garlic is undoubtedly one of the oldest, most widely used foods to fight disease. And with good reason. Since the beginning of the century there have been two thousand studies on the effectiveness of this pungent, Italian delight. By including modest amounts of garlic in your daily diet, you can reduce your cholesterol, lower blood pressure, and help prevent blood clots, say most diet experts. Furthermore, research suggests that eating garlic may be a good way to prevent cancer. Scientists believe that the same sulfur compounds that give garlic and onions their pungent bite are the ones that fight off disease. The allium sulfides, such as allicin, are particularly potent. Research has shown that two to three fresh cloves of garlic a day over a period of four to twelve weeks can lower total cholesterol by 9 to 15 percent, dangerous LDL cholesterol by 16 percent, and levels of potentially dangerous blood fats known as triglycerides by 10 to 20 percent.

Carotenoids—Carrots and sweet potatoes get their unmistakable hues from carotenoids. They're also abundant in other bright red, yellow, or orange fruits and vegetables, as well as in dark green leafy vegetables (where the green chlorophyll masks their lighter hues). They might even be one of the best things plant foods have to offer. The most famous carotenoid, beta-carotene, received some bad press when researchers found that beta-carotene supplements provided no benefit and possibly made things worse for people at high risk for lung cancer. However, diet therapists claim that people who eat the highest amounts of carotenoids from *natural foods* rather than supplements are significantly less likely to suffer a host of ills, including heart disease, cancer, and many more.

Carotenoids work by acting as antioxidants, which means they block the effects of harmful oxygen molecules called free radicals, before they can damage the body. The carotenoid–cancer studies have been particularly promising. One study compared the diets of 368 women with endometrial cancer with the diets of 713 women without cancer. Researchers found that the women who consumed the most beta-carotene had one-half the risk of cancer as those who consumed the least. In a study on lung cancer, researchers from Yale and the Utah Cancer Center found that among 824 people, those who ate the most fruits and vegetables reduced their risk for lung cancer by 40 percent, and those who ate high amounts of beta-carotene specifically cut their risk by 30 percent. And in a study that found that pizza really can be good for you, Harvard researchers discovered that men who ate at least ten servings a week of tomato-based foods reduced their risk for developing prostate cancer by about 45 percent. That's because tomatoes and tomato-based foods are a rich source of a carotenoid known as lycopene, which many scientists believe has a unique ability to fight prostate cancer.

Studies show that carotenoids not only can knock out cancer, but also can keep your heart from missing a beat. In one European study, researchers found that men with the lowest levels of beta-carotene were 78 percent more likely to experience a heart attack than those with the highest levels. Carotenoids can be particularly useful if you're at high risk for heart disease, according to research. One study tracked the diet and health of 1,899 men with high cholesterol for thirteen years. Researchers found that during this period, the subjects who ate the highest levels of carotenoids were 60 percent less likely to have a heart attack than were those who ate the lowest levels.

Finally, you have doubtless heard the joke about carrots being good for your eyes because you never see a rabbit wearing glasses. Research has found that carrots really do keep eyesight clear and sharp, and so do all leafy greens. Boston researchers found that among 800 volunteers, aged fifty-five to eighty-eight, the more spinach and collard greens people ate, the lower their risk of age-related macular degeneration—the leading cause of blindness among people over sixty-five. The protective effects are due to the carotenoids lutein and zeaxanthin, which are abundant in these leafy greens, say researchers.

Flavonoids—Do you ever wonder why the French can chow down all those buttery croissants, smoke cigarettes, smother their entrees with rich cream sauces, and still be half as likely as Americans are to get heart disease? The answer seems to lie in the red wine the French drink and in the fruits and vegetables they eat—or, more specifically, in all the flavonoids those foods contain.

Foods such as onions, apples, and red grapes (including red wine and grape juice) are filled with color crystals known as flavonoids. Research has found that flavonoids dramatically lower the risk of heart disease among people who eat them in abundance.

Finnish researchers who studied more than five thousand men and women for more than twenty years found that those who ate the most of these protective compounds had the lowest risk of heart disease. The Finns who ate the most onions—a good source of flavonoids—cut their risk by 26 percent. And those eating the most apples—another great flavonoid food—reduced their risk by 19 percent.

Lignans and isoflavonoids—Because of the enormous size of the baby boom generation, an increasing number of women are entering menopause. The need to relieve uncomfortable symptoms such as hot flashes is stronger than ever. If you listen to diet therapists, it may be just the time for women in the West to try what their sisters in the Far East have sworn by for centuries—soy.

Soy foods, like soybeans and foods that contain them, such as tofu, tempeh, and miso, are rich sources of lignans and isoflavonoids, which actually mimic the female sex hormone estrogen. An excess of estrogen is believed to contribute to women's health problems, such as breast cancer and menopause symptoms. Lignans and isoflavonoids (phytoestrogens) have the unique ability to attach themselves to some of the estrogen receptors in the body, so excess human estrogen is flushed from your system. Studies in Japan have found that the traditional Japanese diet raises phytoestrogen levels in women to fifteen to twenty times those of American women. As a result, Japanese women have fewer estrogen surges than their American counterparts over their lifetimes and have a much lower risk for breast cancer.

Interestingly, while phytoestrogens effectively lower the body's levels of harmful estrogen, they seemingly supply enough of the healthful hormone to act as hormone replacement therapy for some women. In addition, researchers at the Bowman Gray School of Medicine found that in animal studies, soy was able to lower dangerous LDL cholesterol while boosting levels of healthful high-density lipoproteins (HDL) cholesterol.

Soy also seems equally good for men. Studies show that estrogen inhibits prostate cancer cells in animals, and researchers believe that phytoestrogens can provide the same kind of protection. Researchers point to Japanese men, who have exceptionally low rates of prostate cancer, and who also eat more soy foods than men in most other cultures.

A Wide Variety

Although carotenoids, flavonoids, and phytoestrogens are important, they're not the only protective compounds found in foods. There are many other disease-fighting phytochemicals. The sulforaphane in cruciferous vegetables like broccoli can fight cancer. The polyphenols in green tea are reportedly twenty times more effective as an antioxidant than vitamin C. And hot peppers contain a compound called capsaicin that not only sets your tongue on fire, but also can quench the pain of arthritis.

There are also the simple benefits of all the essential vitamins and minerals that plant foods provide—nutrients that are hard to get from animal-based foods and that most Americans should consume in greater quantities.

Diet experts urge people to eat a wide variety of fruits and vegetables daily because of the unique disease-fighting capabilities in these foods that we've only begun to tap. As a general rule, experts recommend eating a diet composed of at least two-thirds plant foods to one-third or less animal foods. Also, be as colorful as possible, say diet therapists. By making sure you get at least three different colored vegetables or fruits at both lunch and dinner, you will help ensure your optimum exposure to vital nutrients and compounds.

What to Expect

Because practitioners of diet or nutrition therapy range so widely, the types of advice or examinations each would give would vary as well. Whereas some might tout the standard food pyramid information discussed earlier in this chapter, others might direct you toward a combination of therapies, including naturopathic treatments (designed to help your body heal itself in a holistic way), or to supplements of the herbal and organic food variety. Many advocates of this alternative care believe that everyone should consult a professional for diet therapy advice. Specifically, a visit to a diet therapist will be particularly helpful if you have a nagging chronic condition such as allergies, and especially if you suffer from a digestive problem such as an irritable bowel. Also, diet therapy can prevent heart disease and cancer.

FOR MORE INFORMATION

To find a diet therapist close to your home, try contacting the following organization.

American Association of Naturopathic Physicians
601 Valley St., Suite 105
Seattle, Washington 98109
206-298-0126
206-298-0125 (Referral)

ENVIRONMENTAL
MEDICINE

A Different Kind of Homesick

On a typical morning, you get up, take a shower, grab a bowl of cereal, toss down a hot cup of coffee, brush your teeth, put on makeup, deodorant, and hair spray, get dressed, and maybe fill up the tank on the way to your job inside a closed building. And along the way, you've exposed yourself to hundreds, maybe thousands, of insecticides, herbicides, food additives, petroleum products, gas, plastics, and other chemicals that many doctors believe may be harmful.

That's the major thrust of environmental medicine—focusing on the relationship between disease and the various factors in your environment, or what you are exposed to every day. Doctors in this field believe that many of the minor, common ailments we combat daily, such as allergies, asthma, fatigue, and colitis, as well as major league health foes like cancer, all can be traced to allergens and pollutants in our environment. These doctors point to the thousands of people killed by substances such as asbestos as proof that harmful toxins can exist in the environment for decades before they're recognized and removed.

For years, mainstream medical physicians turned up their noses at environmental medicine. They contended that environmental regulations ensure that the environment is rid of overtly unsafe substances. And, pointing to clinical studies, they insisted that it would take phenomenal doses of any one element or trace toxin to make a person sick. What critics weren't counting on is the sheer volume of these substances in our daily environment, how these substances act together, and their cumulative effect over time. The Environmental Protection Agency has identified more than 400 toxic chemicals that have been found in human tissue samples.

Cumulative Effects

Recently, scientists have discovered that many of the agents in our environment have a synergistic effect. That means that while two chemicals may not pose any harm individually, when mixed, their effects often become toxic. Furthermore, not only can combined agents be much more harmful, but one toxic chemical can reduce your ability to fight off the effects of others. For instance, if your body is busy trying to protect your lungs from the harmful effects of radon gas, it probably won't be able to protect them from an assault of second-hand cigarette smoke or smog. Some people are also genetically sensitive to certain substances and are more likely to get sick if exposed to them. Scientists point out, for example, that you may have a genetic predisposition for lung cancer, but you probably won't get the disease unless you smoke or are exposed to air pollutants or irritants. Factors such as poor nutrition and stress can also leave you more vulnerable to the effects of environmental toxins.

Another factor that mainstream medicine hasn't taken into account is lifetime exposure. Although you may not be exposed to much of any one element in a single day, by the time you reach eighty you can accumulate enough exposure to toxins such as lead, which accumulates in the body, for the consequences to be significant. Some environmental medicine practitioners are particularly concerned about the health plight facing America's rapidly growing population of senior citizens because older people tend to spend more time inside. This increases their exposure to indoor air pollutants such as carbon monoxide from gas appliances, fumes from paints and polishes, and formaldehyde from new carpets, drapes, and furnishings.

Others who have a higher risk for suffering the effects of a toxic environment are people living in low-income areas. Not only does pollution tend to be worse in these areas, but low-income people are less likely to get the important health protection they need from eating a nutritious diet or from receiving high-quality medical care.

As the evidence for environmentally triggered diseases mounts, so does the number of physicians who are taking up the cause. In fact, the Institute of Medicine has released a report on environmental medicine calling for all medical students to be educated about environmental and occupational causes of disease.

Environmental Diseases

There are almost as many diseases that can be attributed to environmental causes as there are diseases, according to the practitioners of environmental medicine. The most common symptoms of environmental sensitivity are allergic reactions such as asthma, eczema, hives, itching, red eyes, sore throat, and congestion. But certainly, many other illnesses such as headaches, arthritis, fatigue, colitis, attention deficit disorder, various forms of cancer, and a host of other common, elusive conditions may be brought on by harmful substances in the environment. Following are a few diseases that are receiving the bulk of attention.

Allergies—An unusual sensitivity to pollen, mold, dust, certain foods, food additives, and preservatives, as well as to chemicals such as pesticides, petroleum products, household cleaners, perfumes, and gasoline can wreak havoc on your health. People with allergies may get rashes or headaches. Some people even develop chronic lung troubles. Through a series of tests, a doctor of environmental medicine can help you identify if something in particular is harming you.

Cancer—A woman's chance of developing breast cancer has risen from one in twenty in 1960 to nearly one in eight today. Though about 30 percent of cases are linked to heredity or poor diet, many environmental physicians believe that a large portion of the other 70 percent can be connected to other, likely environmental, sources. A study by New York University found that women with the highest concentrations of chlorinated pesticides, known as organochlorines, in their blood and fat had breast cancer risks four to ten times higher than women with low levels. Furthermore, the World Health Organization has stated that there is a definite link between environmental toxins and pollution and the current increase in cancer rates.

Environmental factors are being linked especially to hormone-related cancers such as those found in the breast, ovaries, testicles, and prostate gland. Various studies have shown connections between chemical pollutants, such as pesticides, fungicides, and insecticides, and breast cancer, endometriosis, and low sperm counts. Even chemicals used in common plastics, everything from house siding to food wrap, have been connected to hormone disruption.

Environmental medicine researchers continue to study how chemicals can create hormone imbalances and genetic mutations and how those cause various forms of cancer. In the meantime, an environmental doctor can tell you what substances you're being exposed to that could lead to cancer down the road.

Rheumatoid arthritis—The causes and treatment of rheumatoid arthritis remain a mystery to mainstream, conventional medicine. Medication and surgery offer little help. According to environmental medicine practitioners, symptoms of this elusive disease can be alleviated by reducing exposure to highly allergenic foods, chemicals, or other environmental irritants. People with rheumatoid arthritis also frequently suffer from various conditions such as migraine headaches, asthma, and colitis, which offers further evidence that the disease is most likely related to factors in the environment, say experts in environmental medicine.

What to Expect

Determining the environmental cause lurking behind your condition is like looking for a needle in a haystack. The problem is that with so many potential causes, how can you nail down the culprit? The task of a doctor of environmental medicine is a complex one. On a typical first visit, you may be asked a long litany of questions on topics including family history, chemicals you're exposed to every day, geographical locations where you have lived, the environment in which you work, and many more. Such questions help the environmental physician to pinpoint any likely elements that may be hurting your health. Also be prepared to undergo one or more tests.

To test for any sensitivities to foods, pollens, and molds, environmental medicine doctors rely on a number of examinations. Many of these exams involve exposing you to the same substances that the doctor suspects are problematic and seeing if they evoke a reaction. By giving you a shallow injection of an irritant and closely monitoring your reaction, the environmental medicine physician can not only make a diagnosis on the spot, but can also test agents you may be able to use to counteract the effects, if you're unable to avoid the offending substance.

Another technique environmental medicine doctors frequently use is known as elimination. A doctor will often recommend eliminating one or more foods from your diet for a period of at least ten to fourteen days, hoping that in that time your symptoms will clear. A few of the foods that most commonly cause trouble are milk and dairy products, coffee, soy, yeast, wheat, corn, tomatoes, beef, pork, chicken, eggs, peanuts, chocolate, oranges, potatoes, and sugar.

An Ounce of Prevention

One of the most important recent ideas in environmental medicine is that coexisting with those things in the environment that make you sick are things that can keep you well. The following are ways the experts say you can help protect yourself against environmental assaults.

Eat your fruits and veggies. Study after study shows that eating a plant-based, fiber-rich diet can help fend off many of the harmful effects of environmental toxins. In many cases, researchers have found that even the most potent cancer-causing substances can be neutralized by protective vitamins, minerals, and phytochemicals in these healthful foods. A diet rich in fruits and veggies provides protection by helping the immune system run at its best. Conversely, studies show that being deficient in certain vitamins and minerals can increase your susceptibility to pesticides.

Trim your weight. Being overweight leaves you more vulnerable to environmental assaults, say experts. When scientists exposed a group of lean rats and a group of obese rats to cancer-causing toxins, the obese rats were one thousand times more likely than their slim counterparts to develop cancer. So it's important to watch your calorie and fat intake.

Exercise early in the day. Though exercising, period, is more important than when you exercise, it's a good idea to work out in the early morning hours, when ozone and smog levels are low.

Shun the sun. Though the sun is not always considered an "environmental toxin," doctors of environmental medicine routinely caution about the risks of unprotected sun exposure. And many mainstream physicians agree that, with one million new cases of skin cancer being diagnosed each year, their advice is well worth heeding. For optimum protection, use the highest sun protection factor (SPF) sunscreen you can and wear a wide-brimmed hat to keep the rays out.

FOR MORE INFORMATION

If you suspect that something in your water, air, or food is making you ill, you can get more information about environmental medicine and find a qualified environmental medicine doctor by contacting one of the organizations below.

American Academy of Environmental Medicine (AAEM)
10 East Randolph St.
New Hope, Pennsylvania 18938
215-862-4544

National Association of Physicians for the Environment
6410 Rockledge Drive, Suite 412
Bethesda, Maryland 20817
301-571-9791

Human Ecology Action League (HEAL)
P.O. Box 49126
Atlanta, Georgia 30359
404-248-1898

FLOWER REMEDY/
ESSENCE THERAPY

Petal Power

What's the first thing we do when someone is hospitalized, loses a loved one, or suffers an equally trying trauma? We send flowers. Flowers play such an important role in brightening our lives that we routinely spray their essences in our homes and on our bodies; buy floral wallpaper, bed sheets, dresses, and ties; and nurture them in our gardens.

It should come as no surprise that some doctors believe that these vibrant, fragrant plants can have medicinal uses, particularly for healing emotionally based conditions such as depression, insomnia, irritability, headaches, and stress-related fatigue and anxiety. Known as flower remedy or essence therapy, this alternative healing modality has been growing since the late 1970s when it began to catch on in America.

Truth is, no one really knows how flower remedies heal, though scientists are always trying to find out. One theory is that the compounds in flower essences trigger the brain to release neurochemicals that actually alter your emotional state by erasing negative emotions such as anger and anxiety. Then, because your body is free from the harmful effects of these stressful emotions, it is able to concentrate on healing itself, say flower remedy researchers.

The Bach Flower Remedies

The seeds of flower or essence therapy were planted long ago. Ancient peoples, including Egyptians, Romans, Greeks, and American Indians all used flower essences to fight disease. Violets, for example, have been used by herbalists for centuries to treat insomnia, anger, irritability, and emotional heartaches. Then, in the 1930s, an English physician named Edward Bach formalized the practice. He became convinced that negative feelings and thoughts such as fear, anxiety, insecurity, jealousy, anger, and shyness were the underlying causes of many physical diseases. To be healed, said Bach, people didn't need medicine for their symptoms; they needed remedies to fight their angst and stress.

The natural solution, according to Bach, could be found in the essences of the wildflowers he saw growing in the English countryside. He spent the next several years testing these medicinal powerhouses, eventually identifying thirty-eight flowering plants and trees that provided relief from a wide array of emotional and physical ailments. These remedies became known as the Bach Flower Remedies. Although research companies have since developed other similar healing essences, these thirty-eight form the core curriculum that flower remedy/essence therapy students learn today.

The Essence of Healing

Bach was certainly not the first to suggest the power of flowers to heal. He was, however, unique in how he prepared and administered flower remedies.

Traditionally, flower remedies are prepared by picking flowers in the morning, when they are still wet with dew. They are then placed in a bowl of spring water and set in full sunlight. After several hours, the solution is poured into a bottle to the halfway point. The bottle is then filled with brandy to create what is called the Mother Essence. Flower therapists will then dilute this to treat a specific condition.

The concentration of the remedy depends on how severe the condition is. You can take a few drops of the full-strength concentration under the tongue. Or you can pour a quarter of the solution in a glass and fill the rest with water or juice for a sipping remedy. The latter method is particularly effective if you are sensitive to alcohol.

FLOWER REMEDY ALERT

Though considered very safe, flower and essence remedies contain trace amounts of alcohol. Experts advise pregnant women and people who are sensitive to alcohol to be sure to consult their physician before taking any flower remedies.

Of course, it's unlikely that you'll be making your own flower remedies. And frankly, the preparations are best left to professionals. The flowers used in Bach's thirty-eight flower remedies, for example, are not your garden-variety flower bed flowers, such as tulips, daffodils, and daisies. Instead, you'll find century, hornbeam, and rock rose, as well as flowering tree essences like elm, white chestnut, and willow. You can buy reference materials from companies that manufacture flower remedies. This literature will describe which remedies are best for which conditions. As a rule, the fewer remedies you take at one time, the better. But experts say it's okay to combine up to six essences if you have a wide array of conditions to treat.

Finally, if life has dealt you a severe blow, such as a divorce or job loss, you may want to try Bach's emergency stress formula. Sometimes called Five-Flower Formula or Rescue Remedy, this emergency stress formula has been around for about fifty years and is used to provide emotional balance to people in distress. Five-Flower Formula mixes rock rose, clematis, impatiens, cherry plum, and star-of-Bethlehem. Typically, you take four drops under your tongue during a time of crisis. You can also buy the solution in a cream, which allows you to apply it topically to injuries like minor burns and bruises. Although it makes a great adjunct therapy during those times of crisis, Bach's emergency stress formula in no way replaces medical care when you have a physical injury, or counseling and medical care when you are severely depressed.

You can buy flower remedies/essences in some health food stores, or you can order them directly through mail order companies (see For More Information). Expect to pay about ten dollars for a standard 10.5-milliliter bottle, which should last several months if kept stoppered and away from sunlight and heat.

What to Expect

A variety of alternative health care practitioners, from homeopaths and naturopaths to chiropractors and acupuncturists, use flower remedies. Even some mainstream doctors have embraced flower/essence remedies as complementary treatments. It's important, however, to remember that these remedies are not used to treat physical conditions directly but rather the underlying emotional causes of your symptoms. The initial consultation and course of treatment will likely be very different from what you're accustomed to.

When you visit a doctor specializing in flower remedies, don't expect to spend a great deal of time talking about your symptoms. Rather, expect to focus on how you're feeling emotionally. The doctor will want your personality, not your symptom, profile.

Because they work from the inside emotional level to the outside physical ailment, flower remedies often take more time to clear your symptoms than popping a pharmaceutical pill. Depending on how many underlying emotional stresses you have, flower remedies can take anywhere from a couple of weeks to a couple of months to take effect. While that may seem like a long time, proponents promise that the healing process gradually lessens symptoms, so if it works you'll be getting progressively better until a day comes when you realize you don't have your problem anymore.

FOR MORE INFORMATION

To locate a flower remedy practitioner in your area, or to order flower remedies and essences through the mail, try contacting one of the following.

The Flower Essence Society
P.O. Box 459
Nevada City, California 95959
1-800-548-0075

Flower Essence Services
P.O. Box 1769
Nevada City, California 95959
1-800-548-0075

Global Health Alliance
193 Middle Street
Portland, Maine 04101
1-800-548-0075

Pegasus Products, Inc.
P.O. Box 228
Boulder, Colorado 80306
1-800-527-6104

HERBAL THERAPY

Earth's Original Pharmacy

Lest you scoff at the power of herbs to heal, take a close look at the labels of pain relievers and decongestants. Realizing just how many of our everyday drugs and medicines come from herbs sure makes a solid case for herbal therapy. Herbs and compounds derived from herbs have made some of mankind's most powerful drugs for centuries. Though most people don't know it, about one-fourth of all the medications that doctors prescribe today are made with active ingredients that are either derived from or are similar to plant medicines. Aspirin, for instance, is derived from acetylsalicylic acid, which is found in the bark of the white willow tree. In fact, even our most common over-the-counter and home remedies are herb-based. When you have a bad burn, aloe vera comes to your rescue. And a little after-dinner mint is just what the doctor ordered to aid digestion.

During recent years, herbal therapy has become increasing popular. In fact, the annual sale of herbal remedies has topped $1.5 billion, according to the American Botanical Council. But there's still one very big problem. Herbs are considered nutritional supplements, not drugs, by the FDA, which means that makers of herbal products are forbidden from putting therapeutic recommendations on the label. This leaves consumers in a quandary about which herbs to take for which conditions, as well as how much is healthful and how much is harmful. This lack of regulation also means there are a lot of cheap imitations.

Fortunately, many diligent herbalists have dedicated the greater parts of their professional lives to studying and to formulating recommended dosages for dozens of herbs. Currently, the World Health Organization recognizes 119 plant-derived pharmaceutical medicines. The result is a better understanding of which herbs work for which conditions; how they should be taken; and the general actions, side effects, and dangers that accompany plant medicines.

Herbal Healing

Herbs refer to plants or parts of plants such as the leaf, flower, bark, seed, root, and stem. Though certain herbs such as cayenne and ginger are technically considered spices when you cook with them in your kitchen, for medicinal purposes they can be classified as herbs.

It used to be that all medicines were based on natural herbs. Then chemists learned how to isolate the active ingredients in herbs and make them into very potent drugs. Once they learned how to make synthetic simulations of natural compounds, the booming, billion dollar pharmaceutical industry was born. Forget herbs. You can patent drugs.

Unfortunately, what doctors didn't count on as they were doling out these new, fast-acting, super-strong prescription medicines were equally fast-acting, super-strong side effects and sky-high health care costs. It is problems such as these that have drawn many people back to the gentler, slower-acting ways of herbal therapy. That's not to say that herbs never have side effects, but they're generally fewer and less severe. For example, many researchers believe that the herb valerian can be just as effective for beating insomnia as sleeping pills. But unlike sleeping pills, it's not addictive. And, valerian is less expensive.

How do herbs work? Well, the same way medicines do. A long time ago, people observed what animals ate when they weren't well. And they experimented themselves until they discovered the many healing actions of various plants.

What they found was that plants had characteristics much like those we attribute to our medicines today. There are anti-inflammatories, astringents, laxatives, expectorants, diuretics, anti-bacterials, and much, much more. The one main difference, which is important to remember when trying herbal therapy for the first time, is that, unlike drugs, herbs often take a little time to work. Sometimes you have to take an herb for a couple of weeks to feel its effects fully, because it does its healing gradually.

HERBAL ALERT

Herbs can be potent medicines. But they can also be potent poisons. It's important to educate yourself about any herb before taking it. A few can cause irreparable damage, disease, or even death if taken the wrong way. Herbs that are potentially dangerous include chaparral, coltsfoot, comfey (internally), foxglove, pennyroyal (internally), pokeweed, and sassafras. Furthermore, even herbs that are healing for some people can be harmful for others. Always talk to your doctor before beginning an herbal therapy regimen. And pregnant women, people with heart or liver disease, or those with other existing conditions should always get a doctor's okay before taking any kind of herbal remedy.

The following are some of the most common herbs used in herbal therapy and the conditions they treat.

Aloe vera—Derived from a plant in the cactus family, aloe has been used for centuries. Cosmetic manufacturers infuse hand creams, face creams, and shaving creams with the gel from aloe leaves because of its skin-softening abilities. And it's even better to keep on hand to soothe minor burns or sunburns. Aloe contains amino acids, vitamins, and minerals as well as a salicylate substance (like that found in aspirin), which can help reduce inflammation. Finally, aloe has a well-known laxative effect, making aloe vera capsules a useful remedy for constipation. Of course, like any laxative, it should only be taken as directed.

Cayenne—Strange though it may seem, this spicy red pepper known as cayenne or red pepper, can actually help soothe the stomach lining and help in the treatment of ulcers and other gastrointestinal diseases. Cayenne is also useful for stimulating digestion, because it increases the flow of digestive juices. Some herbalists say that taking capsules of this spicy herb can increase and improve circulation, making it useful for treating some headaches and circulatory problems such as cold feet. Finally, if you have sore muscles or painful joints, rubbing them with a cayenne ointment can provide quick relief.

Chamomile—The original sleepy time tea, chamomile, which is derived from the chamomile flower, is frequently taken as a relaxant. Chamomile also works as a gentle aid to digestion. And researchers have found that this herb has anti-inflammatory and anti-infection properties. For that reason, some herbal experts recommend a chamomile extract for in-flammations of the skin, inside the mouth and gums, or even the genital region.

Echinacea—This herb may be the first to surpass conventional over-the-counter drugs as a remedy for colds and flu. Originally used by Native American healers in the treatment of snake bites and skin wounds, echinacea has shown modern American researchers just how potent it can be against infections. Studies show that substances found in the echinacea root can stimulate the production of important immune system cells that protect the body against infections, such as those that cause the common cold. Herbalists still use echinacea to alleviate insect bites, acne, and abscesses.

Ephedra—If you have asthma, allergies, or hay fever, you are probably familiar with the effects of the herb ephedra. Known as ma-huang in China, ephedra has long been used for its ability to constrict blood vessels and dilate the wind-pipe—precisely what you need when you're having trouble breathing due to the inflammation caused by asthma or allergies. Though this is not an herb you should use on your own, it's interesting to consider that extracts from its stem are approved for use in common over-the-counter deconges-tant and bronchial drugs. Note: Ephedra should not be used at all by people with heart disease, high blood pressure, dia-betes, or thyroid disease.

Feverfew—If taken at the first signs of headache, herbal therapy researchers say, feverfew can help stop or reduce the severity of a migraine headache. Scientists believe that the herb's active ingredient, parthenolide, inhibits the release of substances like serotonin and prostaglandins, which can trig-ger migraine headaches. Feverfew also appears to have some anti-inflammatory, as well as some anticlotting properties, which may help in preventing circulatory problems.

Garlic—Garlic may be the king of herbs when it comes to having the most scientific backing. Literally thousands of studies have been conducted on this odorous herb during the past century. Researchers are certain garlic plays a positive role in preventing a host of diseases, including cancer and heart disease. Scientists say that garlic is an antibiotic, an immune system stimulant, and an antifungal (for yeast infec-tions, for instance). It helps improve circulation and lowers triglycerides and artery-clogging LDL cholesterol while increasing good HDL cholesterol. Because of its pungent odor, lots of folks prefer odorless garlic extracts to the real thing, but herbalists and scientists agree that fresh garlic cloves are more effective.

Ginger—If the rocking and rolling motion of planes, trains, and automobiles makes you a little green around the edges, ginger could be the answer. Gingerroot can assuage the nausea associated with motion sickness. But that's not all this zesty root does. Ginger is also useful for improving weak digestion and for increasing circulation. Though you might be most familiar with ginger as it appears in ginger ale, that's not its most potent form. It's more effective to boil gingerroot to make tea, or to buy it in powdered capsules.

Ginkgo—Estimated to be more than 100 million years old, the ginkgo tree may be the oldest living herb species. It may also provide one of the newest herbal treatments for problems such as Alzheimer's disease and atherosclerosis. Extract from the fan-shaped ginkgo leaves has been found to increase blood flowing through the brain and also to help prevent blood platelets from sticking together and clotting, both of which help reduce symptoms of memory loss, ringing in the ears (known as tinnitus), vertigo, and some types of headaches. Ginkgo extract generally comes in capsules.

Ginseng—These days you can find ginseng practically everywhere. It's in iced tea. It's sold in vials in convenience store checkout aisles. And ginseng capsules are readily available in grocery stores. Its popularity is almost directly attributable to the reputation ginseng has earned as an energizer. This Asian root has been used as a gentle stimulant for centuries, and is particularly beneficial for men with fatigue and impotence. Herbalists also recommend ginseng to reduce premenstrual symptoms and hot flashes associated with menopause. Further, researchers are exploring its potential to reduce bad LDL cholesterol and triglycerides while increasing helpful HDL cholesterol. Though it may provide a bit of a pick-me-up when drunk in teas, ginseng is most potent in capsule form.

Goldenseal—Goldenseal is a popular American herb that acts as a powerful liver stimulant, antibacterial, and antifungal. When taken internally, it can help fend off yeast-related infections and gastrointestinal conditions like nausea and indigestion. When applied topically, goldenseal can be beneficial against acne, eczema, and ringworm. Goldenseal was traditionally used to induce labor and should be avoided during pregnancy. (See Herbal Alert, p. 76.)

Gotu kola—Commonly used among East Indian people, gotu kola is known as a longevity herb. Herbalists believe it can act as a brain and memory stimulant. Gotu kola is also a diuretic. It's commonly sold in capsules.

Lemon balm—Plagued by seasonal cold sores? Wipe a little lemon balm on your lips. Research shows that this herb can help herpes outbreaks clear up faster and also prolong the period between outbreaks. Lemon balm is also useful for fighting off bacterial infections as well as for soothing nerves.

Milk thistle—Brimming with a mixture of healing flavonoid derivatives known as silymarin, the milk thistle is an excellent herbal treatment for liver disorders ranging from hepatitis to cirrhosis. Data show milk thistle is so potent, it may actually reverse liver disease.

Nettle—Nettle is used throughout Europe in the treatment of rheumatism, arthritis, eczema, and hay fever. Nettle leaves contain a plant protein that may also help stimulate the immune system. You can also use fresh nettle as a diuretic when you're feeling bloated.

Peppermint—Those after-dinner mints you pop on the way out of the restaurant do more for you than freshen your breath. The cool extract from the peppermint leaf has been used for more than two hundred years as a digestive aid. Peppermint oil helps prevent gassiness and stimulates digestive secretions. Peppermint also can be useful for fighting off bacteria and is often used in balms and ointments.

Saw palmetto—As the problems associated with enlarged prostate glands have become public, the benefits of saw palmetto have become more well known. Long used as a tonic for strengthening the male reproductive system, saw palmetto has been shown to be particularly good for treating enlargement of the prostate gland and its symptoms, which include frequent, sporadic urination.

St. John's Wort—Mother Nature's Prozac may be the best nickname for this up-and-coming herb. Herbalists have traditionally used St. John's Wort as a muscle relaxant to ease menstrual problems. Then they discovered that the herb also acts as a mild tranquilizer to combat problems with depression and insomnia. Today, researchers are finding that for many, St. John's Wort is useful for relieving nervousness and anxiety. Applied topically, this calming herb is also an anti-inflammatory and can speed the healing of wounds, bruises, and minor burns.

Valerian—Say goodnight with a dose of valerian. This European herb is as effective as an over-the-counter sleeping pill, say researchers. But unlike some sleeping aids, valerian is not addictive. Unfortunately, it does have one bad quality. It stinks—literally—which doesn't make for a tasty cup of nighttime tea. Herbal experts generally recommend buying valerian in capsule form to make it easier to swallow.

Witch hazel—You're most likely to find witch hazel extract in a bottle of distilled liquid in people's medicine chests. This astringent herb is mighty useful for treating many topical ailments, from bruises and cuts to varicose veins. It's particularly helpful for easing the discomfort associated with hemorrhoids.

Shapes and Sizes

Herbs often come in a wide variety of forms, including liquids, powders, teas, and tinctures. The following is a quick guide to the most common forms of herbs you'll likely find in your local health food store. You can expect to pay anywhere from five to thirty dollars for most herbal medicines.

Capsules and tablets—It's hard to believe that herbs can be so good for you and yet, depending on the kind, taste so bad. Often they're bitter or very astringent. Capsules are good because they make taking your herbal medicine easy. They also have the benefit of providing herbs in precise dosages. The one downside is that some herbalists don't believe that the active ingredients in herbs are released into your body as effectively with capsules or tablets as with other forms such as oils, teas, and tinctures.

Essential oils—Mostly used for aromatherapy (see p. 10), a few essential oils can be taken internally in very small doses of one or two drops. But it's best to consult an expert in herbal medicine before using concentrated essential oils in this way.

Extracts and tinctures—Extracts and tinctures offer the most bang for your herbal therapy buck, say experts. These concoctions are typically made by soaking fresh herbs in alcohol for a few days to a few weeks. The solution is then bottled and ready for use. Tinctures can be made by mixing a specified number of drops into a little water for drinking. If they're made properly, tinctures have an indefinite shelf life. Herbalists often recommend them because they go directly into the system.

Ointments—Generally made with petroleum jelly or vegetable oils, ointments, balms, and salves are herbal products meant to be applied topically, according to directions. They are most frequently used for skin ailments and other external conditions.

Teas—Conveniently available in tea bags as well as loose leaf, herbal teas are an enjoyable way to take some of the more pleasant-tasting herbs such as peppermint, chamomile, and lemon. Teas generally have milder medicinal effects than more concentrated herbal concoctions. And their warm, gentle comfort makes them go down easy.

Whole herbs—Often you can buy the whole herb, which is the medicinal plant or plant part that has been dried and either cut or powdered. From there you can take them home to make your own teas. Do this by pouring one cup of boiling water over one teaspoon of loose herb. Let the mixture steep for about ten minutes and then drain off the tea using a strainer.

Herbal Shopping

One of the trickiest things about using herbs is buying them. There's such an enormous array of products and such a shortage of information, many would-be consumers are left scratching their heads in the herb aisle.

Reputable magazines and books can be good guides for finding out what kind of herbs to buy, what forms to buy them in, and how much of them to take for any given condition. But it's even better to see an herbalist or an M.D., registered nurse, or naturopathic doctor who specializes in herbal medicine. That way you can ask about proper dosages, possible side effects, and potential interactions the herbs may have with medications you are already taking.

FOR MORE INFORMATION

Though herbal medicine is spreading faster than wild-fire across the country, a good herbalist can be hard to find. To locate one in your area, try contacting one of the following organizations.

American Association of Naturopathic Physicians
601 Valley St., Suite 105
Seattle, Washington 98109
206-298-0126
206-298-0125 (Referral)

The American Herbalists Guild
P.O. Box 1683
Sequel, California 95073

HOMEOPATHY

A Touch of What Ails You

Most of us don't know it, but we practice homeopathy all the time. Our introduction to this alternative medicine practice starts when we receive our first vaccinations as infants and continues as we get shots for allergies and antidotes for bee stings later in life.

Though they may not have called themselves homeopaths, scientists such as Jonas Salk and Louis Pasteur were among the most successful early practitioners. They realized that by giving the body minute amounts of a virus or disease-causing substance, you could trigger the body's immune response to that particular "poison."

That is the basic tenet of homeopathy—like cures like. The term itself is derived from the Greek words for "like suffering." Homeopathic physicians believe that symptoms of disease are signs that your body is trying to rid itself of some offending substance, such as bacteria or a virus. To help the body heal itself, a homeopath will prescribe trace amounts of substances that evoke symptoms similar to the disease to stimulate the body's immune response. If you have a fever, for instance, a homeopathic doctor may recommend taking a mixture based on compounds from hot peppers.

In and Out of Fashion

Homeopathy was founded in the late 1700s by a German doctor named Samuel Hahnemann. Weary of bloodletting and other harsh therapies of the time, Hahnemann began to develop a softer side to medicine. It was his belief that if large amounts of certain substances could cause symptoms in healthy people, then smaller amounts of the same substances should be able to treat those symptoms in a person who is sick. The treatment of malaria sparked this theory.

After several days of taking large doses of quinine—the standard treatment for malaria—Hahnemann found that he began to experience classic symptoms of the disease such as trembling and heart palpitations. When he stopped taking quinine, the symptoms went away. He started testing the reactions that other substances evoked on his own healthy body, and homeopathy was born.

Transplanted to the United States by a student of Hahnemann's in the mid-1820s, homeopathy was popular in America during the first half of the nineteenth century. It gradually fell by the wayside as advances in scientific medicine emerged, enticing doctors to abandon homeopathy for other therapies.

Today, homeopathy is experiencing a European renaissance as well as here at home. In recent years, Americans have spent an average of about $250 million annually on homeopathic remedies. And sales are on the rise. About 23 percent of cold remedies launched in the United States in recent years have been homeopathic.

Homeopathic medicines today include common plant substances including as chamomile, onion, and marigold as well as known poisons such as hemlock, arsenic, and mercury.

Less Is More

If the idea of taking something that can make you sick makes you nervous, you're not alone. Lots of detractors of homeopathy have similar concerns. But if the thought of taking a poison as potent as hemlock sounds frightening, consider this: Homeopathic solutions are extremely diluted. Some are so watered down, they essentially contain none of the active compound. That's right. None. Along with the idea that like cures like, homeopathic physicians believe that less is more. As he found that large doses of homeopathic substances evoked enough symptoms to make you sick, Dr. Hahnemann began to experiment with smaller doses. He came to believe that the effectiveness and strength of a substance actually increases the more it is diluted.

Homeopathic remedies are diluted by factors of ten, with the dilution process being repeated until the desired concentration has been achieved. The solution is then labeled according to dilution. For instance, a remedy marked 6X (X is the Roman numeral for ten), means that one part of the active substance has been diluted with ten parts water and the process has been repeated six times. What remains is a solution that contains one part active ingredient per million parts inactive solution.

HOMEOPATHIC ALERT

As is the case with any condition, if you try homeopathy and your symptoms persist or become worse, see your regular doctor immediately. All therapies do not work for everyone or for all conditions, homeopathic experts say.

The dilution doesn't weaken the solution, say homeopaths. As long as the solution is shaken vigorously with each dilution, the potency remains. Like the imprint you leave on a patch of grass where you've been sitting, the solution holds the mark of the active ingredient.

No matter how many symptoms and conditions you have, a homeopath will likely prescribe only one remedy, though that solution may contain more than one active ingredient. Homeopaths contend that one solution is all that is needed to treat all of a patient's symptoms. If you suffer from asthma, anxiety, and hot flashes caused by menopause, for instance, a homeopath will concoct a remedy that will cover the symptoms of all three conditions.

The Proof Is in the "Proving"

Homeopaths discover their remedies through a process known as "proving." That is, they test herbs, minerals, and other substances to see if they will evoke any useful symptoms. Then, to be considered effective, these remedies need to be tested in the treatment of an actual condition.

Unfortunately, homeopathic remedies are not often tested in the clinical settings or according to the standards we're accustomed to in conventional medicine. In recent years, scientists have reviewed 107 controlled trials and found that 81 of them showed that the homeopathic remedies used were more effective than the "dummy" solutions they were compared against. Still, researchers say the results are difficult to pin down. The biggest problem is that researchers have trouble reproducing the positive results found by one study in another. So the evidence is still a mixed bag.

What It Treats

That said, among the best designed trials, homeopathy seemed most effective at relieving symptoms from hay fever and asthma, diarrhea, migraine, and fibromyalgia.

Asthma—In recent research, homeopathy has shown its mettle against asthma. Homeopathic treatment was about 20 percent more effective than a phony therapy in alleviating the symptoms of allergic asthma patients, according to the pooled results of three studies. After prescribing either a fake solution or a homeopathic treatment to 202 people with allergic asthma, researchers in Scotland and England found that four weeks later people who received the homeopathic remedies had their symptoms drop by about one-third, much better than the 10 percent relief in those receiving the dummy solutions.

Colds and flu—The area in which homeopathy has made the most successful inroads is the treatment of colds and flu. You can buy homeopathic remedies for these ailments at health food stores, as well as some drug and variety stores. Like other over-the-counter treatments, they are approved and regulated by the Food and Drug Administration. Because the treatment you need varies according to the symptoms you have, be sure to check the label carefully to determine which homeopathic preparation is most appropriate for your specific kind of cold symptoms.

COMMON CURES

Arnica (leopard's bane): Bruises.
Arsenicum (arsenic): Flu symptoms, upset stomach, diarrhea, vomiting.
Belladonna (deadly nightshade): Headache, coughing, sore throat, fever.
Ignatia: Grief, depression.
Ipecacuanha (ipecac root): Nausea, bleeding.
Ledem (marsh tea): Puncture wounds, bites and stings.
Nux vomica (poison nut): Hangover.

Diarrhea—In one study, eighty-one Nicaraguan children living with severe diarrhea were given oral rehydration with sodium, potassium, and chloride, plus either a homeopathic or a fake solution. Researchers found that the homeopathic remedy shortened the duration of diarrhea by about one day—or 20 percent more effectively than the phony solution. Though the homeopathic solutions differed for each child, most contained the ingredients podophyllum, chamomilla, or arsenicum album.

The bottom line seems to be that although homeopathy may not always help, it really can't hurt. Even conservative medical organizations generally do not disapprove of trying homeopathy as long as you don't forgo conventional, proven medical treatment for serious conditions or neglect to take proven preventative medical treatments such as immunizations and health screenings.

Who Practices Homeopathy?

Like many alternative remedies, homeopathy is a treatment that can be used by many health care practitioners and integrated into a variety of medical settings. Training courses are coordinated through the National Center for Homeopathy in Alexandria, Virginia. Although only Arizona, Connecticut, and Nevada have licensing boards for homeopathic physicians, about 3,000 individual health care practitioners including medical doctors, osteopathic doctors, dentists, chiropractors, nurses, nurse practitioners, and even veterinarians practice homeopathy. Because any of these professionals can practice homeopathy, be sure they're certified.

What to Expect

Upon visiting a homeopathic practitioner, be prepared to answer lots of questions, many of which may seem to have nothing to do with your condition. What kinds of food do you crave? Do you have problems falling asleep? Are you easily stressed? All of these questions help create a symptom picture for the homeopath, so he or she will be able to create the appropriate mix of ingredients for your symptoms. Because homeopaths have about 2,000 remedies from which to select, you can expect the question list to be long and specific. Expect to spend at least an hour in consultation.

FOR MORE INFORMATION

When choosing a homeopathic practitioner, you should be sure they are licensed through the National Center for Homeopathy. The following organizations can help you find a qualified homeopath close by.

The National Center for Homeopathy
801 North Fairfax, Suite 306
Alexandria, Virginia 22314
703-548-7790

International Foundation for Homeopathy
2366 Eastlake Avenue, East Suite 301
Seattle, Washington 98102
206-324-8230

HYDROTHERAPY

Water Works

You're sore and tired from an afternoon of pulling weeds. What is the first thing you think of? A good hot shower. Burn your finger, and the first place you head is the cold water spigot. Complain of stress and related fatigue in many European countries, and you'll be pointed in the direction of the local spa. Water, after all, is the universal healer.

That is the basic tenet of hydrotherapy. Be it a liquid bath, a vapor sauna, or a solid ice pack, water can help cure what ails you. Hydrotherapy is as old as the oceans themselves. Countless nations and civilizations—including the Egyptians, Greeks, Romans, Hindus, Chinese, Hebrews, and Native Americans—have relied on water for its medicinal powers. Though hydrotherapy has taken a back seat to pharmacy in terms of popular methods of healing, it's making a comeback. And if you look, you can still find centers where water is the healing wellspring.

Modern hydrotherapists use water both externally and internally to relieve a host of conditions, especially pain and stress, but in adjunct therapies to treat ailments ranging from viral infection to heart disease.

The Wonders of Hydration

The most widely accepted use of water as healer is when it is used to hydrate the body. Like apples and aspirin, water holds a legendary place in family-doctor wisdom. Water is essential to all body functions. By drinking water, we "oil" our joints, transport nutrients through our blood, control our temperature, and soften our skin. More than that, water keeps us alive. We take it in and lose some of it daily through normal body functions such as sweating and urinating. But if you lose just 9 to 12 percent of your body's water supply, and you risk death.

For optimum health, the average adult needs at least six to eight cups—forty-eight to sixty-four ounces—of water every day to replenish vital fluids. And that's just for normal activity levels. If you're at all athletic, you're losing much more water a day, and need to drink more. If you're active, count on drinking about a half an ounce of water for every pound of body weight every day. For a 150-pound person, that means seventy-five ounces, or almost ten cups of water a day.

Although you get water from all beverages, sodas, coffee, tea and alcohol don't count because they act as diuretics. Because they make you urinate more frequently, you'll actually end up losing water. Plain water works best.

Types of Treatments

Of course, drinking is just one of dozens of ways that water is used to keep people healthy. Doctors who specialize in hydrotherapy also rely on special baths, showers, compresses, and saunas. As a general rule, hot water is used to relax the body, while cold water stimulates it. Water therapies can also work by increasing circulation or by drawing blood away from inflamed areas. The following is a sampling of some of the most common therapies used by experts in hydrotherapy.

Baths and showers—No one has to tell you how nicely baths and showers can relieve general aches and pains from "overdoing it." But that's just skimming the surface, say hydrotherapists. Hot baths and showers are excellent for relaxing and stimulating the immune system, as well as for alleviating joint pain, constipation, and respiratory problems.

Cold baths and showers can tone the muscles, relieve fever, reduce inflammation, fight fatigue, and stimulate the central nervous system.

In a study on the effectiveness of spa therapy (where the person undergoing the therapy alternates between taking baths and high-pressure showers), French researchers found that among 121 people complaining of low back pain, those receiving the spa therapy not only fared better during the three-week study period, but also needed less medication to control their pain a full six months later. This therapy, believe it or not, also is believed to be effective for preventing and treating heart disease.

Body wrap—Used to flush toxins from your system, body wraps can also help reduce fever and induce sleep. With this treatment, a hydrotherapist wraps your entire body in a cold, wet sheet, which is then covered with a wool blanket. Your feet are kept warm with a hot foot bath or warm blankets. The whole preparation stays in place until your body heats up enough to completely dry the wet sheet. In order to clean environmental pollutants from your system, sometimes the blankets are kept on for an extended period of time to trigger profuse sweating.

Cold friction rub—An invigorating way to help alleviate chronic fatigue syndrome, cold friction rubs can also increase circulation to help heal bronchitis and pneumonia. To do this at home, first take a hot shower or bath. Then dunk a washcloth in cold water and wrap it around your hand. Using a circular motion, energetically rub your other arm, hand, leg, and foot with the washcloth. Then switch hands and rub the other side of the body, finishing up by rubbing your chest and abdomen. Be sure to refresh the washcloth in cold water as necessary. When you're done, dry yourself with the same vigorous circular motion. Your skin should be glowing.

HYDROTHERAPY ALERT

Though water therapy is generally as safe as taking a bath, there are certain people who need to take special precautions when using it, particularly people with diabetes, pregnant women, and people with heart disease. To avoid problems, keep the following caveats in mind.

•Hyperthermia (inducing fever) is potentially hazardous if performed improperly. It should only be done by a trained professional.

•People suffering from eczema, serious skin conditions, or acute heart problems should not try neutral bathing.

•If you have diabetes, do not apply hot treatments to your feet and legs.

•Hot foot baths are not good for people with arteriosclerosis or Buerger's disease.

•Cold water treading and foot baths should be avoided by people with sciatica, pelvic inflammation, rheumatism, bladder problems, or digestive troubles.

•Hot immersion baths and saunas are not recommended for pregnant women or people with heart disease, diabetes, high or low blood pressure, or multiple sclerosis.

•Elderly people and young children should avoid long, hot treatments such as immersion baths or saunas, as they may exhaust their systems.

Cold water treading—This is a great way to exercise for increased immunity and vigor, say hydrotherapists. If you're going to try it at home, it's essential to get some secure handles in your shower first, so you have something to hold on to. After a shower or bath, immerse your feet in cold water and simply march in place for a few minutes. Afterward, rub your feet vigorously with a towel.

Colon irrigation—Colon irrigation is a process that flushes impurities from your system. The best-known form of colon irrigation is the enema, which traditionally has been used to relieve constipation. Other forms of colon irrigation include colonics, which can be performed only by an experienced hydrotherapist because the procedures can be dangerous if done improperly. While an enema only cleanses the lower portion of the colon, colonics involve a procedure where the entire length of the colon is flushed with large amounts of water to eliminate toxins. Enemas, on the other hand, can be performed at home. Begin by purchasing an enema bag from your local pharmacy. Then fill it with a pint to a quart of lukewarm water and lubricate the insertion tube. Hang the bag about three feet above you. Then, while sitting on the toilet, insert the tube about an inch or two into your anus and slowly release the solution. Squeeze your sphincter muscles to hold the solution for a few minutes. Then release it into the toilet.

Foot and hand baths—Foot baths are an excellent way to reduce swelling in your feet and legs. Food servers and others who spend long hours on their feet swear by them. By drawing blood away from troubled areas, hot foot baths are also used to relieve menstrual cramps as well as headaches and head and chest congestion. Soak your feet in comfortably hot water for up to thirty minutes and then give your feet a quick rinse with cold water when you're done. Some hydrotherapists also use hand baths. A hot hand bath can be just what the doctor ordered for hands that are crampy and achy from too much writing, yard work, or other activity.

Hot and cold compresses—If you've ever had a sprain or strain, you know how nice ice can be. Whether you're suffering from a minor trauma or from a flare-up of a common case of tendinitis, cold compresses can help bring down the inflammation and ease the ache. Limit the time you apply cold compresses to no more than twenty minutes at a stretch, however, to prevent damaging your skin.

Conversely, hot compresses applied for about one-half hour to the lower back and legs can be great for treating sciatica. Hot, moist compresses on the pelvis can provide relief from painful menstrual cramps. They also can stimulate the immune system, say hydrotherapists.

Hyperthermia—Available only in clinical settings, hyperthermia is used to deliberately induce fever in people whose bodies are having trouble fending off disease-causing bacteria and viruses. By inducing a controlled fever, hydrotherapists stimulate the immune system to help alleviate the symptoms of a wide variety of conditions—most notably chronic fatigue syndrome, upper respiratory infections, and some conditions associated with AIDS.

Neutral baths—Having some trouble sleeping? Maybe you just need to try immersion. When applying neutral bath therapy, hydrotherapists have you immerse yourself up to your neck in water that is just a few degrees cooler than your natural body temperature for about twenty minutes. Neutral baths are used to relieve menopausal hot flashes, insomnia, rheumatoid arthritis, and general emotional agitation.

Sitz baths—A sitz (from the German word for "sits") bath, in which you immerse yourself up to your pelvis in hot and/or cold water, is one of the most common home remedies for hemorrhoids. They're also used to relieve other types of pelvic discomfort such as menstrual cramps, pain in the ovaries or testicles, vaginal irritations, and anal fissures. Cold sitz baths may also help improve the muscle tone in the pelvis, which may help lessen problems with incontinence, say hydrotherapists. When trying a sitz bath at home, be sure to use a tub or basin that is deep enough so that the water reaches your navel when you sit in it. Then just relax and let the water go to work.

Steam inhalation—Very common in the treatment of common colds and flu, steam inhalation breaks up stuffiness and eases your breathing passages. Though you can buy a vaporizer at most drug stores, you can make your own at home using nothing but water and a boiling pot. Simply bring water to a boil in a pot on the stove. (You can add a drop or two of eucalyptus or wintergreen oil to increase its effectiveness.) Then take the pot off the burner, and let the water sit. At the point that the water is still steaming, but not boiling, drape a towel over your head to catch the steam and hold your head about a foot over the pot, inhaling the vapors.

Whirlpool baths—Found in locker rooms around the country, whirlpool baths are athletes' post-workout wonder. The swirling, pulsing hot water can rehabilitate injured muscles and joints as well as soothe everyday stresses and strains. Physical therapists commonly use whirlpool baths to increase injured patients' circulation.

Hydrotherapy at Home

As you can see, many of these practices are perfect for home use because they require nothing more complicated than a faucet, a bathtub, and a towel. Because some treatments aren't recommended for people with certain conditions, like pregnancy, diabetes, or heart trouble, however, it's best to talk to an expert in hydrotherapy before trying many of these techniques on your own if you have or suspect you have one of these conditions. (See Box: Hydrotherapy Alert.) Though there are several water-therapy clinics throughout the country, there may not be one close to your home. If that's the case, many naturopathic and holistic physicians are also knowledgeable enough in hydrotherapy to get you started.

FOR MORE INFORMATION

For more information about healing with water or where to find a trained hydrotherapist close to you, try contacting one of the following organizations.

American Association of Naturopathic Physicians
601 Valley St, Suite 105
Seattle, Washington 98109
206-298-0126
206-298-0125 (Referral)

Bastyr College Natural Health Clinic
14500 NE Juanita Drive
Bothell, Washington 98011
425-823-1300

National College of Naturopathic Medicine
11231 Southeast Market Street
Portland, Oregon 97216
503-255-4860

Uchee Pines Institute
30 Uchee Pines Road, Suite 75
Seale, Alabama 36975
205-855-4764

HYPNOTHERAPY

"You Are Getting Very Healthy"

If you've never been to a hypnotherapist, you probably have a pretty pat vision of what they do: swing a shiny pocket watch back and forth while saying, "You are getting verrrry sleeeeeeepy." Though the primary mission of hypnotherapy is relaxation, the treatment is quite different from what you see in the movies.

Typically, a hypnotherapist will ask you to relax, focus on your breathing, and practice a form of mental distraction such as counting the stripes on the wallpaper or imagining yourself walking through a field of flowers. Though the procedure often has been regarded as somewhat controversial, the American Medical Association approved it as a valid medical treatment in 1958. Today there are approximately 15,000 doctors who integrate hypnotherapy into their practices.

What It Treats

Pain and anxiety—Though different therapists use hypnosis for different conditions, the most common and most well-documented uses for hypnotherapy are for the control and release of pain and anxiety. Professional hypnotherapists can facilitate pronounced changes in blood pressure, breathing, and the autonomic nervous system. Eventually, patients learn how to control these responses on their own, and are able to apply self-hypnosis in stressful or painful situations.

When it comes to relieving the pain associated with cancer, hypnosis—which takes its name from the Greek word for "sleep"—can be second to none, according to studies. In one multidisciplinary study of experts in the fields of family medicine, social medicine, psychiatry, psychology, public health, nursing, and epidemiology, researchers found strong evidence that hypnosis can alleviate the chronic pain connected with cancer, especially among children. The study also found evidence that hypnosis provided relief from the pain associated with irritable bowel syndrome, tension headaches, and temporomandibular disorder, or TMD.

Though more research is needed, doctors believe that hypnosis provides pain relief by preventing pain impulses from traveling across the brain, so the pain never even enters your consciousness. Moreover, because the pain and the anxiety centers of the brain overlap, hypnosis to relieve pain is good for anxiety, as well.

Dentistry—Though many dentists are wary of hypnosis, viewing it as a sort of quackery, almost 3 percent of dentists use it. They believe it helps their patients find relief from pain, gagging, and anxiety during dental procedures and even oral surgery.

Seizures—Finally, scientists have recently discovered that they can use hypnosis to identify and possibly treat people who have non-epileptic seizures, according to researchers at the Stanford University Medical Center in California. About 20 to 40 percent of people who experience seizures (but not epilepsy) have them in response to extreme psychological distress. By using hypnosis, doctors can show people how to use self-hypnosis to bring on their seizures and then control them.

How Hypnosis Works

Any hypnotist will tell you that all hypnotism is essentially self-hypnotism. This is why you cannot be hypnotized and made to do things you don't, subconsciously or consciously, want to do. The hypnotherapist is a facilitator only—giving suggestions so the patient can slip into the proper state.

To be hypnotized, you must first relax your body. Then you must shift your focus away from distractions in your immediate, external surroundings and onto a narrow, select range of objects or ideas suggested by the hypnotherapist or yourself. It is not uncommon, for instance, for a hypnotist to have you focus your attention on an outdoor scene, a favorite activity, or on something specific like the wallpaper.

HYPNOTHERAPY ALERT

Though hypnotherapy is considered a very safe procedure, the World Health Organization cautions anyone with psychosis, organic psychiatric conditions, or anti-social personality disorders against hypnosis.

There are two types of hypnotic states that you can reach. The first is the superficial hypnotic state, which means that you're accepting suggestions while under hypnosis, but you don't necessarily carry them out once you "come to." The second, and less common, is the somnambulistic state. In the somnambulistic state, when the hypnotist makes suggestions you accept them as fact, and you heed the suggestions that have been made during hypnosis after the treatment is through. This state is the most effective in the fight against chronic pain. Once in this hypnotic state, you will probably experience some physical transformations, such as increased relaxation, heightened senses, increased awareness of your internal sensations, and a decreased awareness of your physical surroundings.

Successful hypnotherapy generally hinges on a strong, trusting rapport between patient and therapist; a safe and comfortable physical environment; and, most importantly, the patient's willingness to be hypnotized. Hypnotherapy is not something that can be done reluctantly or skeptically. One of the biggest obstacles to the effectiveness of hypnotherapy is that individuals vary greatly in their susceptibility.

What to Expect

If you go to a hypnotherapist, you can expect to spend much of the first session talking about your condition, what to expect while in a trance state, and any other concerns you may have. Hypnotherapy sessions generally last from an hour to an hour and a half. The number of sessions you'll need varies depending on your condition, as does the cost.

FOR MORE INFORMATION

For more information on hypnotherapy or to find a hypnotherapist close to your home, try contacting one of the following organizations.

The American Institute of Hypnotherapy
16842 Von Karmar, #475
Irvine, California 92705
714-261-6400

The American Society of Clinical Hypnosis (ASCH)
2300 East Devon Avenue, Suite 291
Des Plaines, Illinois 60018
708-297-3317

International Medical and Dental Hypnotherapy
Association
4110 Edgeland, Suite 800
Royal Oak, Michigan 48073
313-549-5594

IMAGERY

Healing From Your Mind's Eye

You're late for an important meeting. As you wait "stewing" for the too-long traffic light to turn green, you imagine everyone sitting around the table, perturbed that you're not on time. As you picture the scene with increasingly upsetting detail, your heart beats faster, your palms sweat, and you can feel your muscles tighten.

Without meaning to, you've just practiced imagery of the most common, and least productive, kind—worry. We use our imaginations all the time. But as the scenario above illustrates, all too often we use them for the wrong reasons. We conjure up images of worst-case scenarios that can literally make us feel sick.

Now picture yourself curled up in your loved one's arms on the living room sofa on a Sunday morning as the day's first sun rays stream across your face and warm your skin. You give a happy sigh as your muscles start to relax and your heart rate slows.

From anxiety and worry to the happy anticipation of an upcoming vacation, our imaginations have a tremendous effect on our physical responses. And imagery experts say that this type of therapy is our most underutilized healing resource. Properly used, imagery can reduce stress, lower heart rate, control pain, help us prepare for upcoming events, and may even help fight cancer.

The Brain's "Secret Channels"

The idea of using imagery to prevent, control, and cure disease is both New Age and age-old. Four hundred years ago, medical theorists declared that there were vital spirits in the brain that "flocked" to the heart by way of "secret channels." These spirits explained the connections between the mind and the body, they said.

Today, we know that the vagus nerve provides a direct connection from the brain to the thymus gland, which is located directly above the heart cavity—one of the places where disease-fighting white blood cells are made. According to research, mental imagery can increase the production of thymic hormones. In addition, there is an intricate system of pathways from the frontal lobes of the brain, where imagination originates; through the body's emotional center, the limbic system; onward through the hypothalamus, the gland that regulates sleeping, eating, thirst, body temperature, sexual arousal, and immune function; and into the pituitary, which oversees your body's hormones.

It is this system that allows your body to react to experience. And it's the same one that makes imagery so effective, say imagery experts. Like it or not, every passing thought has an effect on your body. Using brain-scanning devices, researchers have found that your optic cortex—the part of the brain that is activated when you see—is also activated when you visualize. Likewise, your auditory cortex is active when you imagine hearing things and your sensory cortex kicks into gear when you imagine feeling things. To get the picture, imagine biting into a lemon wedge. It's the physical reaction to visualization that just made your mouth salivate. As far as your brain is concerned, your imagination is almost as good as the real thing. And if it's good enough for the brain, it just may be good enough for the body, according to imagery experts.

Imagining Good Health

Imagery was actually rather popular until around 1600, when it fell by the wayside for about 300 years. It was resurrected again in 1971 when a radiation oncologist in Los Angeles, O. Carl Simonton, M.D., unearthed this "medieval" technique and began using it to help people with cancer. The results were eye-opening.

Working with more than 150 volunteer cancer patients who had been given no more than a year to live and who were receiving traditional cancer treatment, Dr. Simonton instructed them to imagine their strapping, heroic white blood cells knocking the stuffing out of their cancer cells. Four years later, 40 percent of the volunteers were still alive, and the tumors of 19 percent of those survivors shrank. Further cancer studies have shown that people who use imagery in conjunction with their regular treatments are more relaxed and positive about their therapy than those who do not. Many also report being better able to tolerate the rigors of chemotherapy and radiation treatments.

IMAGERY ALERT

As with any alternative therapy, imagery is not meant to replace the advice of your regular physician. See a doctor for any emergency condition or one that one that is not responding to this alternative practice.

Though more research is needed, some investigators have found that imagery can boost the activity of natural killer cells, your body's front line of defense against health threats like virus-infected cells and tumor cells. This capability would also make imagery a promising treatment for autoimmune diseases such as rheumatoid arthritis, colitis, and lupus.

One condition you can count on imagery to treat is stress. Imagery is at the center of relaxation techniques designed to release brain chemicals that act as your body's natural brain tranquilizers, lowering blood pressure, heart rate, and anxiety levels. By and large, researchers find that these techniques work. Because imagery relaxes the body, doctors specializing in imagery often recommend it for stress-related conditions such as headaches, chronic pain in the neck and back, high blood pressure, spastic colon, and cramping from premenstrual syndrome.

What to Expect

Though many health care providers use imagery in their practices, to learn more about applying the technique in your everyday life, you should begin with a psychiatrist or psychologist who specializes in guided imagery. There are about as many ways to use imagery as you can imagine. Some doctors may ask you to visualize your actual cells at work; others will request that you think up images of animals, fictional characters, or machines that represent the parts of the body you want to control. Ideally, you should pick the method you can relate to most easily.

When battling tumors, for instance, people might imagine that their healthy cells are plump, juicy berries, while their cancerous cells are dried, shriveled pieces of fruit. They might picture their immune system as birds that fly in and pick up and carry away the raisin-like cancer cells, while the rest of the cells flourish. Another common image is that the immune system cells are like silver bullets coming in and annihilating the tumor cells.

Other experts recommend actually personifying your condition and "reasoning" with it. This way, they say, you also have a chance to learn from your condition. If you're plagued by headaches, for example, you might imagine your headache as a gremlin tightening a vice across your temples. Ask the gremlin why he's there and what you can do to make him loosen his grip. He might "tell" you you have had too little sleep, too much junk food, or not enough R & R away from work. Take his advice, and there is a good chance your headaches will subside, experts say.

A Home Session

The best way to initiate an imagery session is to relax. First, lie or sit down in a comfortable, quiet location where you won't be disturbed. The goal is to completely relax your body and your mind so you can concentrate on your images. Try progressive relaxation to start. Begin by flexing and relaxing all of your muscles, starting in your face and working your way down to your toes. Or simply concentrate on relaxation breathing, so that with each breath in you imagine calmness flowing into your body, and with each exhalation, tension, and worry exiting. Imagine the calmness sweeping into every part of your body while you become progressively peaceful.

Once you're relaxed, imagine yourself in a favorite place. It can be a vacation resort or a calm, quiet dinner with friends or family. Or you can concentrate on a soothing sound, like waves, or on a calming color. Whatever your preference, just make sure it's an image that makes you feel safe, secure, and relaxed. If it is at all distracting, you won't be able to concentrate fully on your healing images.

When you are fully relaxed and comfortable with your safe image, slowly focus on the condition you are trying to heal—conjuring up the healing images you've chosen. Don't become anxious if you lose concentration. It's common for images to fade in and out. Just try to focus as best you can on the overall healing images for about fifteen or twenty minutes. When you're finished, slowly bring yourself out of your healing images. Leave your quiet, safe place. And imagine yourself completely healed.

Though imagery can relieve stress almost instantly you can't expect immediate results for all your conditions. Many factors determine the effectiveness of imagery, not the least of which are the severity of your condition, the strength of your images, and your belief in the therapy. Experts agree that for optimum effectiveness, practice is key. In the beginning you should spend about fifteen to twenty minutes a day concentrating on your images. Once you're comfortable with the procedure you can shorten the increments and draw on these visual healing cues throughout the day.

FOR MORE INFORMATION

Though imagery can be a perfect therapy to perform at home by yourself, it's best to learn from a professional, especially if you have a particular condition you would like to treat. To find an expert in your area, call one of the following associations.

The Academy for Guided Imagery
P.O. Box 2070
Mill Valley, California 94942
1-800-726-2070

American Holistic Medical Association
4101 Lake Boone Trail, Suite 201
Raleigh, North Carolina 27607
1-800-878-3373

JUICE THERAPY

Fresh-Squeezed Healing

If there's one message that permeates both alternative and mainstream medicine, it's that eating a diet rich in fruits and vegetables is one of the best things you can do for your health. Yet all too often these healthful foods fall by the wayside in the fast-food line of life.

That's when you should try drinking them to get more. Studies show that fresh fruit and vegetable juices not only can be an invaluable supplement to your diet, but they may also be a viable weapon against such diseases as cancer, urinary tract infection, and arthritis. Juices can also strengthen immunity and aid in the prevention and treatment of many other health conditions.

Put a Tiger in Your Tank
If you ate just a bit more than a pound of carrots a day you'd get ten times the daily vitamin A you need (because carrots are a leading source of beta-carotene, which converts to vitamin A in the body). But let's be realistic. Unless you are Bugs Bunny this probably isn't going to happen. But if you drink the juice, all you need are eight easy ounces.

A few glasses of fruit and vegetable juice a day can do wonders for the average person's diet, say experts who specialize in juice therapy. That's because you can get more nutrients from a glass or two of fresh juice than you could ever get from the foods alone, mainly because it's practically impossible to eat that much. The vitamins and minerals are often more accessible in juices than they are in the whole foods—because juicing frees up nutrients that are often trapped in the fiber of the food. You can think of juices as the ultimate vitamin and mineral supplements, say juice experts.

Juices contain more than just vitamins and minerals. They also contain hundreds of phytochemicals, substances which have incredible healing power. Scientists agree that the more phytochemicals you consume in your diet, the lower your risk for serious conditions such as cancer and heart disease. By drinking fruit and vegetable juices you can vastly increase your intake of those important compounds.

Remember, however, that juices are a supplement to the diet, not a substitution. Though fruit and vegetable juices are nutrient-packed, they lack the fiber of the whole foods. Because Westerners already get only about one-half of the dietary fiber they need each day, it is important to keep eating as well as drinking fruits and vegetables.

JUICE THERAPY ALERT

If you are contemplating a juice fast, please do so under the supervision of a specialist if you plan a fast lasting longer than one day. Underlying conditions such as hypoglycemia may jeopardize your health if the fast is extended for longer than this time period. Also, as noted earlier, juicing is not meant to replace normal intake of solid foods.

What It Treats

Plant extracts have been used as healing tonics for centuries. According to juice specialists, fruit and vegetable juices have similar powers. And studies are showing that the specialists are right. Following are some common conditions and the juices that treat them. (Note: None of the juices are meant to replace any medication you currently may be taking, unless cleared by your doctor.)

Blood clotting—Heart attacks occur when blood clots stick to the fatty deposits on the walls of the heart's arteries. Drinking eight to ten ounces of red or purple grape juice a day can help prevent those clots from forming—maybe even more effectively than aspirin. Researchers have found that red or purple grape juice slows the clotting activity of blood platelets by about 75 percent.

Cigarette smoking—Though positively nothing short of quitting can undo the damage done by cigarette smoke, certain juices can help make smoking a little less damaging. Researchers have found that when cigarette smokers drank eight and one-half ounces of orange juice and just over ten ounces of carrot juice daily for three weeks, they had less free-radical damage to their bad LDL cholesterol than periods when they weren't drinking the juices. And, according to researchers, it's free-radical damage to your LDL cholesterol that causes it to adhere to your artery walls, which promotes hardening of the arteries and high blood pressure.

Constipation—You already know what prunes can do for constipation, but prune juice can be even better to get you going again. Prunes contain several compounds, including dihydroxyphenylisatin, chlorogenic acid, caffeic acid, and sorbitol, all of which scientists believe can stimulate the bowel. Half a cup of prune juice—the amount from about four prunes—can help ease your constipation. Don't like prunes? Apples are another good source of sorbitol, and juice experts say that real apple juice can act as a gentle laxative.

Gout—The purines in foods like pork, organ meats, and anchovies can lead to a painful case of gout. Purines are substances in food that cause too much uric acid in the body. Uric acid excess leads to the formation of tiny crystals that lodge in joints and lead to gout. The juice of cherries can cut those purines off at the pass, therefore cherry juice is a traditional treatment for gout.

High cholesterol—Studies show that a couple of cloves of fresh garlic a day can lower cholesterol as effectively as can medication. Because it might be difficult to eat a couple of cloves a day, try adding their juice to other vegetable drinks throughout the day. Then follow up with some fresh parsley juice to help eliminate the odor, say juice experts.

Hypertension—Cantaloupe juice is just brimming with potassium, which doctors prescribe to put the brakes on high blood pressure (though you certainly should not try using it instead of your high blood pressure medication). In addition, cantaloupe and garlic are excellent blood thinners, which also can help to reduce high blood pressure. Although you surely don't want to drink garlic juice straight, it can be a punchy addition to a vegetable juice cocktail.

Motion sickness—No surprises here. People have been using ginger to quiet a queasy stomach for centuries. Ginger juice is excellent for calming motion sickness. And you don't need a lot. The juice from a quarter- to a half-inch slice—diluted with another drink—should do the trick.

Ulcers—Though it shouldn't replace your doctor's prescribed treatment for your ulcer, cabbage juice is an ancient remedy for the pain of ulcers. Cabbage contains a lot of glutamine, an amino acid that has been shown to heal ulcers, according to juice therapists.

Urinary tract infection—Cranberry juice has long been used as a home remedy to fend off urinary tract infections. Now scientists have found that the juice of these tart berries, as well as that of their sweeter siblings, blueberries, can indeed help prevent recurrent urinary tract infections. Studies show that cranberry juice contains a compound that actually acts like Teflon for the bladder—preventing infection-causing bacteria from adhering to the bladder walls.

Researchers say that one-half cup of cranberry or blueberry juice a day at the first signs of infection can keep trouble at bay.

The Fast Track to Health

Though it's a controversial practice, some health experts believe that the best thing you can do with fruit and vegetable juices is to replace your food with them for one to three days—what therapists call a juice fast. Some doctors believe that juice fasts boost your body's natural healing abilities by providing necessary nutrients, while not bogging your body down with lots of food to digest. Your body can take the energy and the hours that it normally devotes to food processing and use them for repairing itself. Plus, your body has a chance to clean house, flushing out all of your stored toxins, say experts. Specialists in juice therapy advise such fasts for a wide variety of conditions, including arthritis, cancer, and AIDS.

Another common use for juice fasting is to detect and eliminate food sensitivities, which some doctors believe are major contributors to immune system disorders such as arthritis, asthma, and chronic fatigue syndrome. Often people with these conditions notice their symptoms lift after a few days of going without food, say doctors who practice juice therapy. Then, when they begin eating the aggravating foods again, their symptoms reappear. A juice fast can be an excellent way to pinpoint and eliminate foods to which you may unknowingly be allergic. Some common troublemakers include corn, wheat, potatoes, and tomatoes, say experts.

Getting Started

Unless you live right next to a juice bar, plan to make some up-front investments to get you started. The most important tool for juice therapy is a juicer. The fruit and vegetable juices you buy at the supermarket have been pasteurized to destroy bacteria and maximize shelf life. The process kills the bad stuff, but, unfortunately it also wipes out many nutrients and enzymes, robbing the juices of any of their therapeutic benefits. Juice therapy practitioners recommend either buying fruit and vegetable juices freshly made from a health food store, or better yet, juicing them yourself right before you drink them to maximize their healthful potential.

THE ULTIMATE VITAMIN AND MINERAL SUPPLEMENTS

Juice experts swear by fresh fruit and vegetable juices to provide the vitamins and minerals you need daily. The following are the major nutrients found in common fruit and vegetable juices.

Beta-carotene: Carrots, cantaloupes, papayas.
Calcium: Kale, collard greens, bok choy.
Chromium: Apples, cabbage, sweet peppers.
Folic acid: Oranges, pineapples, kale, broccoli.
Iron: Prunes.
Manganese: Brussels sprouts, cabbages, turnip greens.
Potassium: Celery, cantaloupes, tomatoes, beets.
Selenium: Apples, turnips, garlic.
Vitamin B6: Kale, spinach, turnips, greens.
Vitamin C: Peppers, citrus fruits, cabbages.
Vitamin E: Asparagus, spinach.
Vitamin K: Broccoli, collard greens, kale.
Zinc: Carrots, ginger, peas.

When purchasing a juicer, look for a machine with the fewest parts. If it isn't easy to use and to clean, you're likely to get discouraged by the hassle every time you want a glass of juice. Depending on the model you buy, you can spend as little as thirty dollars up to as much as a couple of thousand dollars for a juicer. Though you may be tempted by cheaper models, a machine in the $150 to $200 range will serve you best in the long run, say experts. Extracting juice from tough, fibrous vegetables like carrots and beets is hard work that can burn out lesser machines in no time. So, even though the initial investment for a quality machine is higher, you won't need to replace it every couple of years.

If you have never juiced before, be sure to follow the instructions included with your juicer. They will tell you how to peel and prepare your fruits and vegetables for juicing. Most experts also advise using organic fruits and vegetables for your juices to avoid pesticides.

Finally, once you have your freshly prepared juice, drink it up as soon as possible. Unlike pasteurized, commercial juices, the fresh stuff perishes quickly. And, vegetable cocktails—drinks made from two or more vegetables—tend to separate if left standing too long. Fruit juices are the most resilient, but they also lose many of their vital nutrients if left in the refrigerator for more than a day.

FOR MORE INFORMATION

Though some M.D.s have begun to embrace this practice, if you're interested in learning more about using juices to supplement your diet as well as to help cure disease, N.D.s are your best bet. Naturopathic physicians are trained to treat people using a variety of natural methods including homeopathy, herbs, vitamins, nutritional or diet counseling, acupuncture, and, of course, juicing. To find a naturopath in your area, contact the following organization.

American Association of Naturopathic Physicians
601 Valley St., Suite 105
Seattle, Washington 98109
206-296-0126
206-298-0125 (Referral)

LIGHT THERAPY

No Need to Be "Sad"

Most of us go through a period of winter blahs. It's dark when we leave in the morning. It's dark when we come home. It's cold. And it's likely that before the first crocus pokes its head through the newly thawed ground, we'll battle a case or two of the winter blues. For about ten million Americans, however, these blues become deeper than the January snow. They become full-blown depression, or what doctors call seasonal affective disorder (SAD).

People with SAD are generally happiest during the spring and summer. But when the leaves begin to change and the cold weather brings darker, shorter days, their moods change dramatically. They often become moody and have trouble waking up and concentrating. Their energy lags. They frequently binge on carbohydrates and gain weight. Many also find themselves craving cigarettes, caffeine, or alcohol during the winter months. Doctors used to write SAD off as "all in your head." Now they know it's all in your brain. And it can be treated with a simple alternative treatment known as light therapy, which doctors are finding can not only help stave off SAD but may even prevent or ease certain eating disorders and menstrual problems as well.

Let the Light Shine In

To understand how light therapy works, you have to understand what happens each time you open your peepers. When natural light enters your eye, it's converted into electrical impulses that travel along your optic nerve into your brain. Once there, these impulses trigger the brain's hypothalamus gland to send out chemical messengers known as neurotransmitters, which regulate some body functions such as blood pressure, body temperature, breathing, digestion, sexual function, mood, immunity, and circadian rhythm.

Shut yourself off from natural light and you risk throwing all of these vital functions into disarray. For very sensitive individuals, that's exactly what the short days of winter do. Though indoor lighting at workplaces or shopping malls may seem like a reasonable solution, light therapists have found that most artificial lighting, such as fluorescent or incandescent, does not contain the full spectrum of wavelengths. Therefore, it doesn't behave the way full-spectrum natural light does inside the brain. Some scientists believe that receiving sunlight is the only way you can maintain optimum memory, learning, creativity, and motivation, not to mention the motor functions of coordination and balance.

LIGHT THERAPY ALERT

Staring directly into bright lights can damage your eyes. You should always receive instruction from a professional before trying bright-light therapy at home. Tanning beds are not a substitute for light therapy. Finally, though exposure to natural light is important, you still need to protect your skin and sun from dangerous ultraviolet UVA and UVB rays with sunscreen and sunglasses when in the sun for extended periods.

Because most of us don't have the luxury of fleeing to the Florida Keys to soak up more sunlight when we need it, inventive scientists developed machines that simulate the sun. The most common of these creations are the bright-light box and the dawn simulator.

Light boxes are about two feet by two feet in size and contain a bright, full-spectrum light. When using a light box, you should sit about a foot and a half from the screen with the light directed at your face. Then, without looking directly into the light, try to keep your head and eyes exposed to the light while you do other tasks. You could place it on a desk or table while you are reading, eating, or paying bills, for instance. Do this every morning or evening for between thirty minutes and two hours, and you should feel improvements within a week, say light therapists.

Scientists in Switzerland discovered that they could greatly reduce depressive symptoms in twenty-seven out of thirty-nine volunteers with SAD by having them use bright-light therapy for an hour either in the morning after rising or in the evening before going to bed.

The other technique involves using dawn simulators, which are exactly as they sound—machines that trick your body into believing the sun has risen. They work by slowly lighting your bedroom the way daylight would. Because your eyelids are translucent, this simulated sunlight can enter your body while you sleep and help keep your circadian rhythm on track, so you awake feeling alert and rested instead of sluggish and depressed.

You can buy bright-light boxes and dawn simulators through specialty distributors, but it's best to go to a medical practitioner for a referral first so they can help you determine which system is best for you and instruct you on the proper use for your condition.

Not Only for Moods

Light therapy is so effective against SAD that scientists have been testing its potential power against other conditions that may also be triggered or aggravated by brain chemical changes.

Eating disorders—One such condition is bulimia, which is an eating disorder that involves binging on large amounts of food, followed by a purging, either through vomiting or using laxatives. The condition is often connected to depression. Some scientists have found that by increasing levels of the brain chemical serotonin—which also regulates your appetite—with bright-light therapy, they could reduce the number of binge-purge episodes by about one-half.

Menstrual discomfort—Another intriguing possibility for light therapy involves menstruation. Some researchers believe that they can shorten and regulate the menstrual cycles of women who have long or irregular cycles by normalizing their bodily rhythms through bright-light therapy.

Other—Over the years, scientists have been experimenting with the healing powers of many forms of light, including ultraviolet light for autoimmune disease like lupus, and for chronic skin conditions like psoriasis. Some scientists even are investigating the use of light photons to shrink cancer tumors. But much more research is needed before we'll know for sure just how many conditions light can improve.

FOR MORE INFORMATION

Because light therapy is still a long way away from becoming mainstream, you may have trouble finding a doctor who is knowledgeable about the treatment. A psychiatrist or psychologist may be able to point you in the right direction. The following organizations can help you find information on light therapy, and may be able to help you find a practitioner in your area.

Environmental Health & Light Research Institute
16057 Tampa Palms Boulevard, Suite 227
Tampa, Florida 33647
1-800-544-4878

MASSAGE

Rubbing the Right Way

When Swedish fencing master Peter Hendrik Ling came up with a systematic series of muscle rubbing and maneuvering known as Swedish massage, he started a healing revolution in the modern Western world. But massage is hardly new. In fact, it's probably one of the oldest healing therapies around. Artifacts more than five thousand years old show that people in Egypt, Rome, Greece, China, and Japan took healing matters into their own hands. The father of medicine, Hippocrates, wrote, "The physician must be experienced in many things, but most assuredly in rubbing." Today Americans spend an average of $2 billion to $4 billion a year on massage, and some insurance companies are even starting to foot the bill.

Unfortunately, the thought of getting massaged rubs some folks the wrong way. That's because there are some illegitimate businesses operating under the guise of massage, when what they're really offering is "adult entertainment." The American Massage Therapy Association (AMTA), as well as other pioneering people and organizations, work to make sure that all you need to do is look for the right certification to know that you'll be getting the right kind of rubdown from your massage therapist.

Much More than Muscles

Massage is the kneading, stroking, and manipulation of the soft tissues of your body, which include your skin, muscles, tendons, and ligaments. The obvious benefit is relief from muscle tension, but studies show that's not even the half of it. Done properly, massage can also provide better flexibility, improve circulation, lower blood pressure, relieve headaches, improve posture, strengthen the immune system, reduce stress, and more. The following are some of the common conditions that can be relieved by massage, according to researchers and others.

Asthma—Stress is a recognized trigger of attacks among asthma sufferers, and because massage is such a great stress-reliever it only makes sense that massage may be good for preventing asthma attacks. In one small study, seventeen out of nineteen people with asthma noticed an improvement in their symptoms during a three-month period of weekly half-hour massage sessions.

Muscle soreness—If you are at all active, you'll find that regular massage therapy can enable you to recover more quickly from injury. It also reduces the likelihood of further injury, increases flexibility, and helps reduce muscle soreness related to exercise and activity.

Pregnancy-related discomfort—Researchers have found that during the first trimester of pregnancy, massage can relieve headaches as well as reduce morning sickness, nausea, and fatigue. During the second trimester, it can alleviate back pain and leg cramps. Massage in the third trimester is helpful in fighting pregnancy-related insomnia and swelling. And some practitioners believe that by improving blood flow, massage can help prevent anemia during pregnancy.

Premature birth—In a study that shows you're never too young to benefit from massage therapy, researchers at the Touch Research Institute at the University of Miami School of Medicine found that premature babies given three fifteen-minute massages a day gained 47 percent more weight and were discharged an average of six days earlier than infants who did not receive massage therapy.

Stress—Studies clearly show that massage can alleviate stress of all kinds. In one study from the Touch Research Institute at the University of Miami School of Medicine, researchers found that when healthy adults were given a fifteen-minute chair massage in their office twice a week over a five-year period, they not only reported less stress and anxiety, but also were more alert and had improved performance with math problems. As a result of findings such as this, more than 100 large companies, including Adolph Coors, American Airlines, and General Motors, have begun to offer on-site massage to decrease the stress and increase the productivity of their workers.

MASSAGE ALERT

Pleasant and healing as a massage can be, if you have a medical condition you should get your doctor's okay before scheduling one. Some medical disorders are strictly hands off. If you have one of the following conditions, you should not have a massage without first consulting your physician, according to the American Massage Therapy Association:
- Heart disease or high blood pressure
- Infections or open wounds
- Contagious skin disease or rashes
- Phlebitis or circulatory problems
- Cancer
- Serious sprain or strain. (You should wait about forty-eight hours for inflammation to go down before having the area manipulated.)

Elbow Grease

Though there are countless kinds of massage, each employs some common techniques for manipulating your muscles and soft tissues. Expect a therapist to use his or her elbows as well as forearms, hands, and fingertips to get the job done. Your massage therapist should also use a good lubricant like mineral oil to reduce friction and create a smooth, slightly slippery surface to promote effective massage strokes. The following massage techniques are the most common.

Friction—Friction involves the use of your fingertips and thumbs to work deep circles into the thickest part of the muscles and around the joints. This technique is effective for working out hard knots in muscle tissue as well as making joints more flexible.

Kneading—Sometimes called compression or *petrissage,* this technique closely resembles what you do with baking dough. Therapists use their fingers, palms, or thumbs to grasp a muscle, lightly pull it up away from the bone, and roll and squeeze it before releasing it and repeating the process. Like stroking, kneading increases circulation. Kneading is also useful for clearing out any built-up lactic acid, the muscle by-product that gives you that achy feeling the day after you exercise.

Percussion—Also called *tapotement,* percussion alternates between using gentle tapping, chopping, or striking movements with the hands. Therapists use short bursts of percussion both to invigorate and stimulate your muscles. Conversely, they'll sometimes use long bouts of percussion to tire out a muscle and cause it to relax, which is particularly useful for crampy muscles.

Stroking—Also known as *effleurage,* massage strokes are commonly slow and rhythmic and are performed using fingertips, palms, thumbs, or knuckles. Stroking is generally a warm-up technique and it is used to improve circulation.

Vibration—With this technique, the therapist employs fingers or flattened hands to jostle, or shake back and forth, an entire muscle for a few seconds. Vibration is what is used to increase circulation as well as improve the function of your glands and nervous system.

From the West

One of the most popular massage forms in the United States today is the Swedish massage. Not generally employed as a deep muscle massage, Swedish massage involves the use of long strokes, kneading, and friction of the superficial layers of muscle. The therapist strokes in the direction of the heart. And he or she also may lift your appendages to gently work your joints through their range of motion.

Swedish massage is used mostly to improve circulation and increase muscle relaxation. Therapists believe that Swedish massage also stretches out contracted muscles and releases built-up toxins in the muscle tissue that clog up and obstruct the flow of lymph and blood. Though Swedish massage is a full-body treatment, it is especially helpful for sore back and neck muscles.

A form of massage therapy related to Swedish massage is deep tissue massage. As the name implies, this form uses more hand pressure and works deeper into the muscle than its Swedish ancestor. Deep tissue massage either follows or goes against the grain of the muscle. And it can be used for either specific trouble areas or for full-body tension relief.

From the East

Similar to acupressure, shiatsu, which literally means finger pressure, is the Eastern world's answer to the deep muscle massage of the West. Actually, shiatsu probably came first, say experts, considering that Chinese traditional medicine has been applying pressure to special healing points all along the body for about five thousand years.

Shiatsu massage therapists use the tips of their fingers, and sometimes even their elbows and feet, to press and massage special points on the body known as acupoints. These are points along a system of meridians in the body that traditional oriental medicine philosophers believe transfer life energy, or qi (pronounced "chee"), throughout the body. (For more on acupoints, see Acupuncture and Acupressure on p. 1). Practitioners believe that stress can create blockages along these channels, causing physical discomfort or even disease. Shiatsu massage is meant to clear these blockages and promote healing and general well-being.

Though not all Western practitioners agree on the philosophy of meridians and qi, Western research suggests that pressing on acupressure points does in fact trigger the release of endorphins, which act as the body's natural pain killers.

What to Expect

It's natural to feel apprehensive the first time you go for a massage. Because of the intimate nature of the therapy, it is important to be entirely at ease with your massage therapist. And he or she will certainly do everything possible to make your experience a comfortable and rewarding one.

First, expect to answer questions much like those you'd receive from any medical professional or therapist. You'll likely be asked about your reasons for wanting a massage, your current physical condition, medical history, lifestyle, any areas that are painful or achy, the nature of your work, your stress levels, and other pertinent topics.

Once the massage therapist is ready to begin your session, you'll be asked to undress in private and wrap yourself with a towel, sheet, or gown that the therapist will provide. If it makes you more comfortable, you are perfectly welcome to leave on your undergarments. During your massage, you'll be lying down on a massage table, covered up except for the areas that the therapist is working on.

The environment should be peaceful and pleasant. Many therapists will use incense, calming music, and fragrant oils. If at any point any smell, sound, or sensation is troubling you, you should feel free to tell your therapist. Also, you and your therapist should discuss the level of physical discomfort you expect as well as the difference between a "good hurt" and a "bad hurt" before you start. You should leave feeling better, not beaten up.

Most massage sessions last thirty to sixty minutes and can cost from twenty to seventy dollars an hour, depending upon where you go.

FOR MORE INFORMATION

When seeking a qualified massage therapist, make sure they have one of the following three credentials: Certified Massage Therapist, Licensed Massage Therapist, or Registered Massage Therapist. Contact the American Massage Therapy Association (AMTA) to help you find a qualified professional close to home.

American Massage Therapy Association
820 Davis Street, Suite 100
Evanston, Illinois 60201-4444
847-864-0123

NATUROPATHY

All Nature's Cures Wrapped up in One

Visiting a naturopathic physician is like seeing a half-dozen alternative healers at the same time. Grounded in the concept that your body is its own best healer, naturopathic physicians are trained in clinical nutrition, herbal medicine, hydrotherapy, homeopathy, acupuncture, bodywork, light therapy, sound therapy, and lifestyle modification—all intended to help you better heal yourself.

Naturopathy is more than a system of medicine; it is a system of living. The naturopath prescribes a way of life that treats the person instead of the condition or disease from which you are suffering. The basic tenet is that health and vitality are your natural state of being and that nature is your best physician. By combining your body's ability to cure itself with healing agents found in nature, naturopaths believe that you can maintain good health throughout your entire life and avoid the common deterioration that we have come to associate with aging.

Naturopathic medicine was founded by Benedict Lust in Germany in 1892. Eventually, he opened the American School of Naturopathy in 1907. Unfortunately, by the middle of the 1930s, naturopathic medicine was elbowed aside by our high-tech modern system. Currently, naturopathy is enjoying a resurgence as people seek more holistic, natural healing methods. Today many states allow naturopaths to be trained and licensed by following a similar educational path as conventional doctors. Some can even prescribe medication, and insurance companies are increasingly likely to cover some naturopathic treatments.

What It Treats

Like many alternative medicines, naturopathy excels in the areas where modern medicine often fails—in the treatment of chronic conditions such as allergies and arthritis. It also can be the perfect complementary treatment for diseases such as cancer, hypertension, and cardiovascular disease. In fact, there are few, if any, diseases that would not respond to naturopathic care—either as a primary treatment or as complementary therapy to quicken the healing and recovery process.

NATUROPATHY ALERT

Serious medical conditions like heart attack, as well as traumas from accidents and injuries, require conventional medical treatment. Naturopathy is beneficial for helping quicken recovery from these conditions and for the treatment of chronic diseases and minor ailments. Always consult with your physician before beginning a new course of treatment.

What to Expect

Because there are so many modalities involved in naturopathy, you will find a wide variety of treatment styles among naturopathic physicians. Some pay heed to natural healing methods only, for instance, while others practice a medical style similar to that practiced by conventional doctors, except that they employ some alternative techniques to quicken the healing process. The underlying principles are the same. The style you choose is up to you.

Expect to spend about an hour at your initial visit with a naturopathic physician. Naturopaths want to know about everything in your life that can affect your health. This includes questions about your medical history, diet, environment, exercise habits, stress, lifestyle, exposure to toxins, health habits, and your mental and emotional status. Like conventional physicians, the naturopath may also ask you to take the typical gamut of tests including blood work, X-rays, and a urinalysis.

Naturopaths follow a system of healing that begins with purging you of your bad habits and ends with teaching you new ways to take responsibility for your health. The following are the principles of naturopathic living as they were explained by Lust.

Eliminate bad habits. Naturopathic physicians say you can't have your cake and eat it, too. If you want good health, you need to get rid of some decidedly unhealthy habits. For optimum health and vitality, naturopathic doctors recommend ridding yourself of alcohol, drugs, and caffeine as well as negative emotions such as worry. They also suggest that people get out of the habits of skimping on sleep and wasting their vital energy on excessive sexual intercourse.

Learn healing habits. Once you've dumped your bad habits, naturopaths focus on teaching you new habits that promote health. These include proper breathing, appropriate daily exercise, a healthy mental attitude, and moderation in work and play.

Practice naturopathic principles of living. Living naturopathically means adopting some new lifestyle practices. Fasting, mud baths, bodywork, organic eating, steam baths, and other healing practices become part of your daily life.

Eat naturopathically. Naturopathic practitioners focus on eating a diet based on organically grown, whole foods. But that's just scratching the surface. Naturopathy teaches that everyone is biochemically unique, and that we each have specific dietary needs for optimum health. It's your naturopathic physician's job to help you determine the best diet for your constitution.

Let the body heal itself whenever possible. Naturopaths believe that the body has the ability to heal itself. Often they will let a fever or inflammation run its course if it doesn't become health threatening. They suggest that people not overdo antibiotics and other medicines for minor conditions, but rather let the body heal itself when it can.

Unfortunately, even if you do everything right, you will occasionally collide with toxins in your environment that cause disease. For these times, naturopathy also has a specific approach to healing. The following are the principles of naturopathic medicine.

Use the healing power of nature. Above all, naturopaths believe that nature knows best. When you're sick, the naturopath's job is to use all of the natural remedies at his or her disposal, from soft tissue manipulation to botanical preparations to facilitate the healing powers of the body.

First, do no harm. Hippocrates said it first. Naturopaths vow to live by it. Whenever possible, naturopathic physicians use noninvasive treatments with minimal side effects. They rely on effective, natural therapies and are trained to know when a disease is out of their scope of practice and when to refer to another health care provider.

Treat the cause, not the symptom. If you have a fever, naturopathy teaches that you should treat the thing causing your fever, not the fever itself. Every illness has an underlying cause—generally a problem with diet or lifestyle habits. It is the naturopath's job to locate and remove those factors so the disease is not only cured—it doesn't recur.

Treat the whole person. You are more than what you eat or how you think. You are a complex mixture of physical, mental, emotional, spiritual, genetic, and social elements.

Naturopathy teaches that you need to take the whole person into account for effective healing. Some diseases that appear untreatable by physical standards, for instance, may respond to spiritual healing, according to the laws of naturopathy.

Practice prevention. Naturopathic physicians aim to keep you well. The goal is not only to prevent disease in the first place, but also to prevent minor ailments from becoming major degenerative diseases.

Establish wellness. Those who practice naturopathic medicine believe that wellness exists within all of us, regardless of what diseases may be present at any given time. They strive to tap into your source of wellness so that you're inherently strong enough to heal more quickly from onslaughts of disease than you would through treatment alone.

View your doctor as your teacher. You must take responsibility for your own health, according to the tenets of naturopathic medicine. The doctor exists primarily to teach you how to best take care of yourself.

Bringing It All Together

The treatments that naturopaths employ when treating disease are every bit as multifaceted as the diseases themselves. Nowhere in naturopathic medicine will you simply walk out with a prescription for pills and a recommendation to call if you get worse.

Generally, the naturopath will initiate treatment with acupuncture or homeopathy to start the wheels of healing in motion. Then he or she will use dietary recommendations, botanical supplements, and vitamin and mineral regimens to bolster the body's healing systems that are flagging under the burden of disease. Depending on your condition, the naturopathic practitioner may also employ hydrotherapy, massage, and bodywork, as well as light and sound therapy to restore the body's natural healing ability. There are some naturopathic physicians who are also certified to perform certain surgical treatments such as suturing lacerations, performing skin biopsies or hemorrhoid surgery, setting fractures, and other minor procedures that may become necessary.

Finally, the naturopathic physician will try to locate and eliminate any emotional or spiritual disharmony that may be causing or contributing to the disease process. You can look to your naturopathic doctor for guidance in establishing harmony in these areas of your life. They are often trained in psychology and personal and family counseling as well as physical healing.

Because naturopaths are not yet licensed in all states, it is important to check the background and accreditation of your practitioner to ensure he or she has formal training. Three naturopathic schools exist in the United States: the National College of Naturopathic Medicine, Bastyr University, and the Southwest College of Naturopathic Medicine and Health Science. Ask where your practitioner was schooled before making an appointment.

Because not all states recognize naturopaths as primary care providers, you should also check with your insurance company about its reimbursement policies.

FOR MORE INFORMATION

To find a qualified naturopathic physician in your area, try the following organization.

American Association of Naturopathic Physicians
601 Valley St., Suite 105
Seattle, Washington 98109
206-298-0126
206-298-0125 (Referral)

OSTEOPATHY

Home-Grown Healing

During the mid-nineteenth century, a Methodist minister, Andrew Taylor, needed a way to care for his parishioners' physical, as well as their emotional and spiritual needs. His answer was osteopathy, a medical system that takes conventional medicine a few steps further—using spinal adjustment and other manipulative approaches to help the body heal.

Similar to chiropractors, osteopaths believe that manipulating the spine can have powerful effects on the rest of the body. They also contend that most diseases have underlying musculoskeletal causes. According to osteopathic philosophy, one of the most common causes of health problems is a condition known as "subluxation," or the shifting of a vertebra out of position, causing the one directly below or above it to move out of position in the opposite direction.

Like budding conventional allopathic (modern medicine) doctors (M.D.s), osteopathic medical students study basic anatomy and physiology. They sit through all the same lectures and labs. But clinical medical training begins earlier for osteopathic students because osteopaths need to put in 200 hours of hands-on training in osteopathic manipulation.

The end result is that osteopathic physicians provide a true melding of conventional and alternative medicine. Generally, they will treat patients using traditional allopathic techniques until the condition calls for something above and beyond conventional medicine. Then, they will apply osteopathic manipulation.

What to Expect

To determine whether or not a patient requires some type of musculoskeletal manipulation, osteopathic doctors focus on symptoms different from those examined by traditional doctors. Mostly, they are looking for any mechanical problems within your body.

Expect your osteopathic physician to inspect your posture or gait to see how you hold yourself while standing, sitting, and moving around. He or she will see whether you have any problems moving your joints through their full range of motion. The osteopath also will check your body's symmetry and will inspect your muscles and joints for any irregularities such as fluid retention, slow reflexes, or tenderness. If the doctor suspects serious pathology, he or she will likely call for some conventional screening techniques such as X-rays, blood tests, and MRIs.

OSTEOPATHY ALERT

Spinal and limb manipulation is not beneficial for every condition (in fact, it can even be downright harmful). Fortunately, osteopathic physicians are trained in conventional as well as osteopathic therapies, so they not only know when manipulation is inappropriate, but they can treat the condition through other means.

If your osteopath decides that you would benefit from physical manipulation, he or she will use one or more of a series of techniques to bring you back to a balanced state. Here are some of the most common manipulation approaches.

Articulation. This is a quick thrusting movement the osteopath uses to shock the body into proper position when your motion is severely limited.

Cranial manipulation—A subtle, gentle approach used to slightly manipulate the skull bones and stimulate the production of brain hormones.

Functional and positional release—Here, practitioners place you in a position that allows your body to relax and work through muscle spasms that have resulted from injury.

Mobilization—The practitioner gently moves a joint through its full range of motion to eliminate any restrictions in movement.

Muscle energy treatment—Patients are asked to constrict and then relax specific muscles throughout their bodies.

Osteopathic practitioners, recognizing that no individual treatment works in a vacuum, frequently employ relaxation techniques, breathing exercises, nutritional counseling, and exercise recommendations along with their in-office treatment. And they will likely refer you to a bodywork specialist, such as someone trained in the Alexander technique or Feldenkrais, to help you learn and maintain proper posture and to prevent you from needing major future adjustments.

What It Treats

As mentioned, osteopathic doctors don't use their bone-manipulation techniques for every condition. Generally, they reserve them for treating underlying structural or postural problems that may be causing back pain, neck pain, conditions like sciatica and arthritis, or some kinds of respiratory problems. Research also supports osteopathic treatment for chronic fatigue syndrome, high blood pressure, allergies, headaches, and some symptoms of PMS.

Though osteopaths don't typically use manipulation for all conditions, they believe that most, if not all, conditions can benefit to some degree from the effects of osteopathic manipulation. When your posture is corrected, your joints are free from constriction, and your spine is straight. Your body responds with improved circulation, boosted immune function, and a healthy nerve supply to organs and tissues. All of the above promote healing, say osteopathic physicians.

Though osteopathic treatment traditionally has been restricted to spine and limb manipulation, some experts are moving into the controversial area of osteopathic manipulation of the bones in the skull. About 100 years ago, a few osteopaths suggested that by ever-so-gently manipulating the seemingly immobile bones that make up the cranium, you could trigger the release of important brain hormones. Others said it could not be done. Today, experts generally agree that if the doctor has strong-enough hands, he or she can indeed cause the skull bones to shift very slightly along their divisions. The idea has some osteopathic psychiatrists hopeful that by combining cranial manipulation with traditional treatment they may be able to bring about quicker, more lasting results.

Another experimental area of osteopathic care to keep an eye on is known as "somatoemotional release." Here, osteopathic physicians are attempting to treat emotional problems by manipulating different body regions they believe have connections to those emotional centers. It's too early to tell how effective it may be, but research is currently underway.

The Doctor Is In

Unlike many struggling alternative therapies, osteopathy has come a long way in gaining respect in the mainstream health community. In the past, the rivalry between medical doctors (M.D.s) and doctors of osteopathy (D.O.s) was one of bitter disrespect. But these days osteopathic doctors are just as likely as their allopathic colleagues to hold positions of high esteem in major medical institutions across the country.

Osteopathic medicine is making major inroads throughout Europe, as well. Several years ago the Osteopath's Bill was signed, making osteopathic the first alternative health care system to receive legal recognition in Europe.

In the United States, you have your pick of about 35,000 doctors of osteopathy who carry the same licensing and practice parameters as medical doctors. You can also expect to pay about as much for treatment sessions with an osteopath as you would for treatment from an M.D. Fortunately, most major insurance companies should help foot the bill. Call yours to be sure.

FOR MORE INFORMATION

Unlike many alternative health therapies, it should be relatively easy to find a licensed osteopathic practitioner close to your home. But if you run into trouble, one of the following organizations can help.

American Academy of Osteopathy
3500 DePauw Boulevard
Suite 1080
Indianapolis, Indiana 46268
317-879-1881

American Osteopathic Association
142 East Ontario Street
Chicago, Illinois 60611
312-280-5800

SOUND THERAPY

Music to Heal By

Every time you turn up your favorite tunes while cruising down the highway, you're practicing sound therapy. When you play some soft Mozart for a special candlelit night, that's sound therapy, too. In fact, though, there's certainly more to sound therapy than spinning your favorite CDs. Most of us practice some form of sound therapy each day of our lives, whether we mean to or not.

When you think about how everyday sounds affect our moods and well-being, it's not so hard to accept the theory that sound can heal. Imagine, for instance, that you're in a room with a crying baby, a hair dryer, and a staticky radio. Got a headache already? Okay, now go to another room filled with the soft sound of ocean waves breaking, flute music playing on the radio, and coffee percolating on the stove. Feel your blood pressure drop? Doctors today believe sound, especially music, has healing powers.

English Restoration playwright William Congreve said it best when he penned the immortal words: "Music has charms to soothe a savage beast. To soften rocks, or bend a knotted oak." Dentists caught on much later when, in the 1930s, they began to use music to complement the less-than-perfect anesthesia of the time. Today, treating adults and children with emotional disturbances is the biggest area for sound therapy, though its use is spreading into many treatments, including those for Alzheimer's disease, stress, heart disease, sleep disorders, and more.

The Science of Sound

To understand how sound or music therapy can heal, it helps to know what happens when sound enters your body. Some researchers believe that there are particular physiological reflexes that respond reflexively to music. For instance, music can influence your heart rate, blood pressure, skin temperature, gastrointestinal function, eye pupil size, muscle tension, brain wave activity, and immunity.

Remember, sound is energy. It's technically known as "oscillating energy waves within an audible range." And music is nothing more than sound waves arranged in a pleasing sequence. When these sound waves enter the ear, they travel to the brain through the eighth and tenth cranial nerves. From there, motor and sensory impulses are sent along the vagus nerve, which is partly responsible for regulating breathing, speech, and heart rate. The impulses travel to the heart, larynx, throat, and diaphragm. Some researchers believe that it is this connection as well as the vagus nerve's connection to the limbic system (the system believed to be responsible for human emotion) that enables sound and music to be a powerful healer.

Researchers have found that music can increase the production of your body's natural pain-killers—endorphins—as well as affect your internal rhythms. This is why your heartbeat speeds up when you hear the cadence of a marching band, or slows down to shopping mall piped-in music.

Another growing theory on the healing power of sound is that sound waves can directly affect individual components within the body. The therapy grounded in this theory is called "cymatic" and is used by holistic doctors in some parts of the United States. This treatment is based on the scientific fact that every single atom vibrates, emitting sound waves that the human ear can't hear. Because we're made up entirely of atoms, our cells make these inaudible sounds, too. Some practitioners believe that stress or sickness can alter these sound waves, making your health condition worse. These practitioners believe you can encourage healing by directing sound waves at the cells that are being affected to restore their natural rhythm.

Alternative doctors who follow Far Eastern philosophies also believe that sound heals by balancing the body's energy centers, which are known in Eastern medicine as *chakras*. There are seven chakras, which can be thrown out of rhythm by stress and disease, say some doctors. By applying the rhythm of music, they believe, these chakras can be returned to their appropriate rhythms, which helps the body to heal.

Finally, and most simply, music can be a pleasant distraction during otherwise stressful medical procedures, say experts. Generally speaking, when selecting music for healing, you want to reach for soothing rather than stimulating tunes. Experts recommend selecting compositions that are played at sixty beats per minute or less, which, as you might guess, means more classical music than rock and roll. Good choices include music by the classical composers Johann Sebastian Bach, George Frideric Handel, and Georg Philipp Telemann. New Age music also works very well, as much of it is written with the express purpose of stimulating one's relaxation and healing.

What It Treats

Though research in this field is still relatively new, there's a large body of scientific proof that sound or music therapy can be effective for a variety of conditions. Music has already been well established to help ease stress. Here are some other well-researched areas in which it may be helpful.

Alzheimer's disease—Music therapy is making exciting headway into treatment of Alzheimer's disease. Researchers find that familiar music not only can tap into the memories of Alzheimer's sufferers, but also that it may decrease related agitated and aggressive behavior.

Investigators believe that music therapy may be capable of decreasing levels of ACTH, cortisol, and catecholamine in people who have Alzheimer's disease while simultaneously increasing levels of endorphins, serotonin, and other calming, pain-relieving brain chemicals. Studies conducted so far have been positive.

Colds—Researchers at Wilkes University in Wilkes-Barre, Pennsylvania, found that soft music, especially the Muzak you hear while on hold or riding in an elevator, can do more than fill a void while passing the time. It can actually boost your immunity against such conditions as upper-respiratory infections. When the investigators exposed university students to thirty minutes of a particular Muzak tape, their levels of IgA—an antibody that is associated with protection against respiratory infections—increased more than 14 percent. Don't like "elevator music"? Try listening to jazz. When the students listened to smooth jazz, their IgA levels increased over 7 percent.

Pain—Music that appeals to you can reduce pain—plain and simple. People who visit hospitals, gynecological and obstetrical centers, surgical centers, and dentist offices where music therapy is applied report less pain and more positive feelings about their experience than those who visit centers without music therapy. Some people report feeling more relaxed and even needing less anesthesia during procedures.

Sleep disorders—Older adults often have trouble falling asleep and getting enough sleep. Research shows that music therapy can help. In one study from the University of Louisville, researchers gave twenty-five volunteers with sleep disturbances either New Age or Baroque music to play when they were having trouble with sleep, either at night when they couldn't fall asleep or in the early morning when they would wake up prematurely. All but one of the volunteers reported they slept better when they used music therapy.

Surgery recovery—There seems little doubt that music can help ease the recovery process of people who have recently undergone surgery or who have been hospitalized for treatment. One study compared two groups of postoperative patients for a period of forty-eight hours. One group received music therapy during the recovery time and the other did not. At the end of the study, researchers found that those receiving music therapy had reductions in blood pressure and heart rate. Other doctors have reported that heart surgery patients who use music therapy have fewer complications than generally occur with that type of procedure.

Even listening to music before surgery seems to help. Studies show that people who listen to classical music for about twenty minutes prior to surgery come out of surgery with less post-surgical anxiety than those who do not—probably because they go into surgery with less anxiety, say researchers.

The Maestros of Music Therapy

Though sound therapy might sound as simple as putting six CDs in the changer and hitting "shuffle," there are some conditions that are best put in the hands of a professional. And everyone, no matter what their situation, can benefit from a little instruction before they turn up the volume on music as therapy.

When looking for a qualified expert in music therapy, look for the initials RMT, for Registered Music Therapist; CMT, for Certified Music Therapist; or MT-BC, for Board-Certified Music Therapist. Any of these folks can help you find the music that suits your needs. In addition, trained sound or music therapists integrate a variety of tools into their practice, using musical instruments, tuning forks, tapes, and even machines that emit sound waves at specific frequencies created to heal specific ailments. A music therapist can help you learn how to make your own healing music with advanced musical instruments, singing, or humming.

Often, there are hospitals, rehabilitation centers, and nursing facilities that offer group music therapy, but you can also hire a private music therapist to train you one-on-one for an hourly fee of about fifty dollars, depending upon where you live.

FOR MORE INFORMATION

To find a qualified music therapist in your area, try contacting the following organization.

The American Association of Music Therapy
8455 Colesville Road, Suite 930
Silver Spring, Maryland 20910-3392
301-589-3300

TRADITIONAL
CHINESE MEDICINE

Elemental Healing

Of all the alternative healing modalities, Traditional Chinese Medicine (TCM) may be the most difficult to grasp. When it comes to ideas about the human body, East and West are worlds apart.

TCM is rooted in five-thousand-year-old philosophies that view each patient as his or her own miniature universe. Instead of focusing on disease, doctors of TCM focus on the wellness of a person, believing that disease means that there is imbalance or disharmony within that individual's universe. Therefore, what causes cancer or even a cold in you may be totally different from what causes the same conditions in your neighbor. In short, TCM treats the patient, not the disease. TCM also introduces various elements, such as life force, or *qi* (pronounced "chee"), which Western medicine denies exists. So if you're interested in TCM, be prepared to expand your horizons.

Equal but Opposite Forces

By now, we've all seen the swirling black and white circular symbol of yin and yang—the two polar opposite forces of the universe, according to Eastern philosophy. Yin is the cold, dark, inward-moving facet of the universe. Yang is the light, hot, active, outward-moving quality. One cannot exist without the other. And, ideally, they exist in equal measure.

Unfortunately, the world and the people living in it are rarely so perfect. Practitioners of TCM believe that the underlying cause of all physical conditions is an imbalance of one or the other of these driving forces. When you're running low in yin, for instance, your body's yang takes over, drying you out with its excessive heat and causing symptoms such as constipation, thirst, and dry skin. Conversely, when yang is in short supply, your body's yin runs unchecked and causes symptoms like chills, chronic fatigue, and diarrhea. Every organ in your body is subject to yin and yang imbalance, which TCM practitioners treat with herbs, exercises, acupuncture, and other Chinese healing modalities.

Though balance is the ideal, it's important to realize that people generally have a tendency to fall to one side or the other of the yin-yang spectrum. Therefore, we are all more susceptible to specific conditions that are related to our personal imbalances.

Your Universal Constitution

According to TCM, your body is not a separate entity in this universe, but it is a part of the universe, comprising universal energies, forces, and compositions. Again, a healthy body and mind depend on these forces flowing freely and steadily within your system. The following make up the human constitution, according to TCM.

The force is qi. Qi is the life force in Chinese Medicine. This vital energy flows through a system of fourteen meridians in the body. If one of the meridians becomes blocked, qi can't get through to nourish that part of the body, and you begin suffering symptoms of imbalance, such as mental distress or physical illness. When qi is generally weak all over, you see signs of fatigue, poor appetite, poor digestion, and weak physical constitution. Practitioners of TCM will often prescribe exercises and tonics to increase your qi and thereby improve your well-being.

The essence of Jing. *Jing,* or essence, is responsible for the physical structure of life and your body. It is the fundamental force that is associated with growth, development, and reproduction, and is passed down to us from our parents. We also get it from the food we eat. Excessive sexual activity and stress are jing depleters. Premature aging, early graying of the hair, poor memory, failure to thrive, and conditions affecting bones and teeth such as osteoporosis are blamed on jing that is off-kilter.

Shen lets you be you. *Shen* is what makes you unique. Shen is your mind, your psyche, and the intangible expression of your personality. It's your spirit. Appropriately, shen is believed to be stored in your heart. We nourish our shen through our diet. And when shen is strong we are ripe for good health, strong spirituality, and longevity.

Moisture protects. As you might expect, your body's moisture is made up of the fluids that buffer organs and joints and lubricate your tissues. Moisture is your body's connecting substance.

Blood, a connecting force. TCM does not define blood in the traditional sense. Rather, blood is the substance that forms your bones, nerves, skin, muscles, and organs.

The Five Elements

Just as the earth consists of universal elements, so does your body, according to TCM. These primary elements are fire, earth, metal, water, and wood. Each organ in your body is believed to consist primarily of one of these elements. Just as trees depend on the earth and water to grow, each organ depends upon the others to thrive.

Fire is the element that rules your heart and small intestine. Earth makes up your spleen and stomach. Metal drives your lungs and large intestine. Water is the working element of your kidneys and bladder. And wood is the element that creates your liver and gallbladder.

Your organs are divided into categories of yin and yang. The heart, spleen, lungs, kidney, and liver are considered yin organs because they are thicker and more solid. The small intestine, stomach, large intestine, bladder, and gall bladder are hollow, "carrying" organs that fall into the yang category. The primary yin organs also make up your "organ networks," which govern other parts of your constitution. So you have a heart network, spleen network, lung network, kidney network, and liver network. The following are the domains that each organ network rules, according to the principles of Traditional Chinese Medicine.

The heart network—This network governs shen, arteries, the propulsion of blood, joy, clear perception, and also intuition. When the heart network is out of whack, symptoms such as panic, angina, palpitations, and sleeping problems can result. Overstimulation can disrupt this system.

The spleen network—Spleen is the ruling network over moisture, muscles and flesh, and also thinking and memory. When this system is out of balance, bloating, fatigue, and poor concentration can occur. Too much worrying is often what throws this network off.

The lung network—This network governs qi, skin and hair, circulation and breathing, and also internal drives and appetites. When your lung network is not working up to par, you may experience tightness in the chest, skin rashes, colds and flu, and melancholy. Grief disturbs this network.

The kidney network—This network oversees jing, bones, the brain, and instincts. A troubled kidney network can result in stunted growth, infertility, low back pain, paranoia, apathy, and despair. Overworking yourself and being pessimistic can cause problems in this network.

The liver network—Blood, tendons and nerves, qi, and blood pressure and volume as well as an individual's temperament and judgment fall under the jurisdiction of the liver network. Muscle tension, high blood pressure, head-aches, moodiness, and cramping result when the liver net-work is not working well. The cause of the problem is often anger and frustration.

TCM ALERT

Just because something is alleged to be an ancient Chinese remedy doesn't mean it's good, or that it's safe. Quackery knows no bounds, international or otherwise. Products such as Chinese ma huang, sold in stores as Herbal Ecstasy or Cloud 9, sickened more than four hundred people and killed fifteen before the FDA banned it for potentially causing heart attacks, strokes, and seizures. Some over-the-counter herbal preparations have also been found to contain poisonous compounds like mercury and lead. Be sure to buy and use TCM herbal products under the supervision of a trained TCM professional.

Taking Your Temperature

When the outside elements act upon the elements that make up your body, you are also susceptible to certain conditions. Heat, coldness, dampness, dryness, and wind are often the culprits when you feel out-of-sorts.

Too much heat is responsible for such conditions as constipation, inflammation, irritability, fever, and indigestion. Too much cold causes diarrhea, achy joints, low blood pressure, and poor digestion. Too much dampness can bring on nausea, lack of appetite, and watery stools. Excessive dryness can result in dehydration, dry skin, raspy cough, and dry stools. And high amounts of wind can make you susceptible to vertigo, instability, and trembling.

Again, a trained practitioner of TCM recognizes the underlying elemental causes of such conditions and prescribes treatment to counterbalance the offsetting effects of these universal elements.

Herbal Treatments

Doctors of TCM rarely just prescribe one treatment modality to cure a person suffering from symptoms of a disease. Rather, they use diet therapy, acupuncture, exercise, and, most importantly, herbal therapy.

In Asian countries such as China, doctors prescribe herbal preparations like we prescribe medications. *Kampo*, or Chinese herbal medicines, are a growing phenomenon in many countries, but especially Japan, where they account for the U.S. equivalent of $56 billion in drug sales. Proponents of TCM believe that herbal remedies are preferable to Western-type medications because they provide the healing agent in its natural environment rather than in an isolated form. They believe that by extracting the healing element from the other components in the plant, you set yourself up for all the side effects we typically see in medications because the other compounds in the plant provide balancing and buffering effects.

There are too many herbs to cover them all. But ones you may find familiar are ginseng, astragalus, ginger, and dong quai. Herbs are extracted from bark, roots, leaves, and all parts of plants of all kinds. A professional TCM practitioner generally combines several herbs and administers them through a variety of techniques including pills, powders, syrups, suppositories, soaks, salves, inhalants, and tinctures.

In recent years, many common TCM herbal preparations have been put to the test by Western researchers, and in many instances have come through with flying colors. Because of the intricate and precise ways that herbs must be combined so as to interact with your organ systems, you should only take herbal preparations under the care of a trained expert in TCM.

Qigong Self-Care

Qigong is perhaps TCM's most simple self-help therapy. It is a set of mental and physical exercises that promote spiritual and physical benefits. In China today, experts estimate that some 200 million people practice this energizing exercise every day.

Proponents say that qigong can prevent everything from colds to cancer, which, of course, hasn't been proven. But studies both here and abroad do show that when practiced regularly, qigong can reduce stress, increase circulation, and help your body fight disease. The following are some sample qigong exercises. Remember when you do them that they are most effective if you relax and take your time.

Massage your meridians. Rub your hands together to warm them and increase qi. Then start at your face and stroke your palms upward over your cheeks, eyes, and forehead. Next, rub the side of your head, down the back of your neck, and along your shoulders. Follow your body with your hands beneath your arms, down your ribs, around to your back, across your buttocks, and down the back and sides of your legs all the way down to your feet. Then move around to the top and front of your feet, up the front of your legs, up the front of your torso, and back to your face.

Breathe in the qi. Start in a standing posture with your feet about shoulder-width apart. Relax your body and mind. Then inhale slowly. While you breathe in, let your arms stretch out and float up to shoulder height straight in front of you, keeping your elbows slightly bent. As you exhale, straighten and stretch your arms out. Then as you start inhaling again, let your arms bend slightly and drop down slowly until your hands fall to the sides of your legs. Repeat for a few minutes.

Twist your waist. Assume the standing position with your feet shoulder-width apart. Hold your arms out from your sides as though making a cross with your body, but don't bring them all the way up to shoulder height. Using your upper torso as the moving force, twist at the waist, moving your shoulders and head along in line. Your arms should be loose enough to swing around so your hands and arms lightly thump against your body with each twist.

What It Treats

Like Western medicine, TCM is used for everything that ails you. Records in America dating back to the mid-nineteenth century show that doctors practicing TCM in Oregon and Idaho successfully treated respiratory, digestive, and reproductive infections, as well as arthritis and symptoms of cardiovascular disease. This ancient health philosophy has developed a strong-enough track record that in the 1960s the World Health Organization supported the dissemination of information about it into developing countries.

Traditional Chinese Medicine is probably best appreciated for its effectiveness against chronic conditions such as asthma, headaches, allergies, high blood pressure, and diabetes. When it comes to treating more serious diseases including cancer and AIDS, TCM is often used in conjunction with modern Western medicine to yield the best results. Though TCM is often too complex and philosophical to be easily studied by Western research criteria, many of its herbal preparations are easily studied, and have been. Here's what research has shown so far.

Alzheimer's disease—Chinese folklore has long held that drinking tea brewed with a type of club moss known as Huperzia serrata can perk up people's memories. Now Western researchers are finding that Huperzia may be effective against Alzheimer's disease. Scientists have found that the compound inhibits acetylcholinesterase—an enzyme that breaks down acetylcholine, a chemical messenger that is key in brain memory and awareness.

Cancer—Even some Western doctors have recently given TCM their approval in the treatment of acute promyelocytic leukemia (APL), a rare blood cancer that can be deadly. Doctors found that a Traditional Chinese Medicine arsenic compound, which has been used for centuries against various maladies, actually was bringing about complete remission in about 70 percent of APL patients. Some remained in complete remission for twenty years. The compound works by inducing the cancer cells to go into a state of apoptosis, or "programmed cell death." More studies are being done.

Eczema—Studies show that herbal therapy has been able to reduce the symptoms of eczema by 60 to 90 percent over the treatment period of a year. But more research is underway to test for possible side effects from long-term exposure to the herbal preparations used to treat eczema.

Infertility and impotence—Researchers are reporting that various herbal concoctions including ginger, ginseng, licorice, and atractylodes, are able to increase sperm concentration and sperm mobility and decrease impotence.

What to Expect

Unlike what we've come to expect from a doctor's visit, an appointment with a doctor of TCM will not involve blood tests, X-rays, endoscopy, or invasive treatments such as exploratory surgery.

What you should expect during an initial visit to a TCM practitioner is a lot of personal inspection. The doctor will inspect your complexion, tongue, general disposition, and demeanor as well as characteristics like the strength and tone of your voice and the smell of your breath and body. The doctor also will interview you about your symptoms, diet, lifestyle, general health, and medical history. Finally, the doctor will check your pulse at your wrists, abdomen, and at certain places along your body's meridians. By cross-checking these factors, a TCM practitioner can make a diagnosis about what is affecting your whole person, not just one or two of your organs.

Because of its whole-person approach, many people turn to Traditional Chinese Medicine to complement their disease-focused health care.

FOR MORE INFORMATION

When looking for an expert in TCM, look for a professional with an OMD (Oriental Medical Doctor) degree or a DOM (Doctor of Oriental Medicine) degree. To find a practicing TCM professional in your area, try one of these organizations.

American Association of Acupuncture and
Oriental Medicine
433 Front Street
Catasauqua, Pennsylvania 18032
610-266-1433

American Foundation of Traditional Chinese
Medicine
505 Beach Street
San Francisco, California 94133
415-776-0502

Qigong Institute/East-West Academy of the
Healing Arts
450 Sutter Street, Suite 916
San Francisco, California 94108
415-788-2227

VITAMIN AND
MINERAL THERAPY

Supplementing Your Health

At the turn of the century, people used to get terribly sick for what seemed like mysterious reasons. Sailors would become ill and often die from a condition that, among other things, would cause tooth decay, extreme fatigue, and bleeding problems. Poor people in the South would often fall victim to a disease that caused diarrhea and dementia. And children in Northern climes would suffer a crippling bone deformity.

What they didn't know then, but we know now, is that all of these diseases have a common cause—vitamin deficiency. Once they started giving lemons and limes to sailors, the vitamin C kept scurvy at bay. Pellagra went away as soon as Southern folks started eating foods filled with niacin. And all that those children living in upper latitudes needed to get back on their feet again was some sunshine to give them their vitamin D.

Scientists learned around 1906 that there are special compounds in foods that people need every day just to stay alive. They called these substances vitamins, meaning "vital for life." In the next three decades, researchers were busy discovering vitamins—assigning each an alphabetical letter as it was discovered. Over time, they discarded those that actually weren't vitamins and added others to the list. (That's why there is no vitamin F, but there are eight vitamin Bs.)

Furthermore, they found a mine of other compounds known as minerals, such as magnesium and sodium, that we all need as well. Together, vitamins and minerals became known as essential nutrients.

In 1941, medical scientists determined the minimal amounts of nutrients people need to prevent deficiency diseases. They called these amounts the Recommended Dietary Allowances (RDAs). Small adjustments were made to these numbers in recent years, and nutritionalists started calling them the Daily Values (DVs).

Daily Values (DVs)

Scientists have since learned that although these minimum amounts may keep us from getting deficiency diseases, they don't necessarily keep us as healthy as we could be. In fact, years spent skating around the lower levels of our nutritional needs might be making us sick. Doctors who practice vitamin and mineral therapy are banking on the notion that we can prolong or avoid many ailments, including heart disease and cancer, by taking in the *optimum* amount of essential nutrients. And studies are backing them up.

The Health Spectrum

The first problem with the DVs is that they aren't specific enough. Though these recommendations make some differentiation between the needs of men and women, they don't reflect the difference in nutritional needs among children, adults, and the elderly. In addition, people who are very active, who smoke, drink alcohol, or who are at high risk for diseases such as osteoporosis have special nutritional needs that these daily recommendations do not consider.

The second problem is the one mentioned earlier. The DVs are based on the minimum amount of nutrients you need just to stay alive. And there's a big difference between being really healthy and being deathly ill. Health is not an all-or-nothing proposition. Between being perfectly healthy and having scurvy is a wide gray area where you don't have the energy you'd like and where your body isn't working as it should. This is where proponents of vitamin and mineral therapy come in. Based on scientific research, they recommend the amounts you should be taking for optimum health. Consider vitamin C, for instance. The DV says you need sixty milligrams. But countless studies show that vitamin C boosts immunity when you take it in doses closer to 200 to 500 milligrams, acting as a real protective force against diseases like cancer, diabetes, and heart attack. Another good example is vitamin E. The DV calls for a quite tiny thirty International Units (IU). Vitamin E researchers will tell you that you need a whole lot more. Most heart disease studies are done using 400 to 1,200 IU of vitamin E—not only many times the DV, but more than you could ever get from food alone.

The FDA is slowly, but surely, recognizing that much higher amounts of essential nutrients may be necessary to prevent degenerative diseases associated with aging, like heart disease, diabetes, and cancer. But it will probably be many years before they can tell you how much. Vitamin and mineral therapists contend that there is no need to wait to reap the benefits of these widely available compounds.

Food or Pill?

The question that always comes up when talking about vitamin and mineral therapy is whether you really need to take vitamin and mineral supplements when you can get them from food. About 100 million Americans think we do need to supplement. They spend more than $4 billion a year on vitamin and mineral supplements. And increasing numbers of nutritionists and doctors, both alternative and mainstream, agree that supplementing your diet with some essential nutrients can be a good idea.

Nutrition experts say that one of the biggest problems we face these days is being both overweight and undernourished.

Much of our food supply is processed "junk" such as white bread, potato chips, and hot dogs. These foods may supply plenty of calories, but they've been stripped of much of their vitamin and mineral content. The United States Department of Agriculture (USDA) has found that though most of us clearly aren't starving, we are still getting less than 70 to 80 percent of the DV we need each day.

You'd have to drink bottles of olive oil or eat jars of mayonnaise to get the 400 IU of vitamin E that doctors advise for preventing heart disease—a decidedly less-healthy alternative to simply taking a vitamin E capsule.

VITAMIN AND MINERAL ALERT

When it comes to vitamins and minerals, you can definitely have too much of a good thing. Taking very high doses of certain nutrients can cause toxic reactions over time. Do not exceed recommended doses of vitamins and minerals without talking to a trained professional first. This applies especially to women who are pregnant and to children.

That said, you should never use vitamin and mineral supplements as a replacement for a healthy diet. Although they can help make sure you get all your essential nutrients, there are hundreds, maybe thousands of other compounds found in foods known as phytochemicals—such as beta-carotene and lycopene—that not only can assist vitamins and minerals in doing their jobs, but also can help fight diseases like cancer. And, of course, there are amino acids, essential fatty acids, and other nutrients beyond all the vitamins and minerals you need as well. You can only get all of these very healthful compounds from a diet filled with plenty of whole grains, fruits, and vegetables.

What You Need

Experts consider about thirteen vitamins and fifteen minerals essential to good health. For clarification, vitamins are organic compounds found in living things, and minerals are nonorganic compounds that are also found in foods, but in much smaller amounts. Though there's a wide range of opinions about what the ideal dietary intakes really are, vitamin and mineral researchers generally agree on the optimum ranges. The following are the essential vitamins and minerals, the amounts leading nutrition experts recommend, and what they're good for. Note: The listed recommendations are for adults only. You should consult with your doctor before giving supplements to children.

VITAMINS

Vitamins are divided into two categories, fat soluble and water soluble. As their names imply, fat-soluble vitamins are dissolved in fat and water-soluble vitamins are dissolved in your body's watery fluids. Because fat-soluble vitamins are stored in your fatty tissues, they are the ones that can cause problems with toxicity. You should not exceed recommended safe dosages when supplementing fat-soluble vitamins.

Fat-Soluble Vitamins

Vitamin A—Vitamin A in its pure form is found in foods such as liver. But you can also get it as beta-carotene (which turns to vitamin A in the body) from bright orange and leafy green vegetables like carrots, spinach, and broccoli. Vitamin A is essential for tissue growth and healing. Studies show it is particularly useful for protecting against infections, preventing eye problems such as cataracts, and possibly fending off cancer. The DV for vitamin A is 5,000 IU. You should look for supplements with that amount, but not more than 10,000 IU.

Vitamin D—It's also known as the sunshine vitamin, because your body converts sunlight into vitamin D. You can also get vitamin D by eating liver or by drinking milk fortified with vitamin D. Because this nutrient's primary job is regulating calcium metabolism so you can form bone, it is important in the prevention of diseases like osteoporosis. The DV for vitamin D is 400 IU. Experts recommend supplementing between 200 and 400 IU a day.

Vitamin E—Found in foods like nuts and seeds, vitamin E is one of the most difficult vitamins to get from food alone. Vitamin E is primarily an antioxidant, meaning that it fights cell-damaging free-radicals, which have been linked to cancer and heart disease. Experts recommend supplementing between 200 and 800 IU daily.

Vitamin K—This little-known vitamin is found in foods such as spinach, broccoli, and dairy products. Vitamin K is essential for healthy blood clotting. There is no official DV for vitamin K, but experts suggest making sure you get about 300 micrograms. A healthy diet should provide plenty of this essential nutrient, but you can supplement fifty micrograms if you wish, say experts.

Water-Soluble Vitamins

Folic acid—Found in oranges, tuna, and strawberries, folic acid is necessary for building red and white blood cells and for growing and repairing. It is used to prevent birth defects and to ease stress and fatigue. The DV for folic acid is 400 micrograms. You should not supplement more than that amount, say experts, as too much folic acid can hide a vitamin B12 deficiency.

Biotin—This B vitamin, found primarily in peanut butter, eggs, and wheat germ, is important for helping the other B vitamins do their jobs and for processing fat, protein, and carbohydrates. It is sometimes used to help regulate blood sugar levels in people with diabetes. The DV is 300 micrograms. You can safely supplement up to 400 micrograms.

Vitamin B1 (thiamine). Found in unprocessed whole grains and pork, thiamine is essential for changing the food you eat into energy. It's also used to treat diarrhea and muscle cramps. The DV is 1.5 milligrams, but it may be a good idea to supplement up to ten milligrams a day, say experts. You should not supplement more than 100 milligrams on a regular basis.

Vitamin B2 (riboflavin)—Found in milk, salmon, and asparagus, riboflavin is necessary for forming red blood cells and for turning fat, protein, and carbohydrates into energy. The DV is 1.7 milligrams, but you can supplement between twenty-five and fifty milligrams safely.

Vitamin B3—(niacin). Found in meat, poultry, fish, and whole grain cereals, niacin is important for healthy nervous system functioning. It is sometimes used to treat high cholesterol. The DV is twenty milligrams, but you can add up to up to 100 milligrams safely, say experts.

Vitamin B5—(pantothenic acid). Found in fish and whole grain cereals, pantothenic acid is another B vitamin that is essential for turning food into energy. It is also used by nutritionists to relieve stress and fatigue. The DV is ten milligrams. Experts say you can safely supplement up to 100 milligrams.

Vitamin B6—Abundant in food sources such as fish, chicken, and soybeans, vitamin B6 is necessary for normal tissue growth and protein metabolism. The DV for vitamin B6 is two milligrams, but higher doses currently are being used to help relieve many conditions, from symptoms of PMS to carpal tunnel syndrome. You can supplement ten to fifteen milligrams safely, say experts.

Vitamin B12—Prevalent almost exclusively in animal foods like milk, meat, and eggs, vitamin B12 is essential for growing new tissue, forming red blood cells, and changing food to energy. It is used in large doses to treat fatigue, especially among the elderly. The DV is six micrograms, though you can supplement ten to twenty micrograms, especially if you don't eat much meat or other animal foods.

Vitamin C—Citrus fruits, bell peppers, and strawberries are good sources of this super antioxidant nutrient. Vitamin C is essential for building blood vessels and healthy skin tissue, as well as for squelching cell-damaging, disease-causing free-radicals. Vitamin C is used for a wide array of conditions, but most commonly as treatment for and prevention of the common cold. The DV is sixty milligrams, but experts often recommend supplementing anywhere between 300 and 3,000 milligrams.

MINERALS

Calcium—Remember Mom telling you to drink your milk for strong bones and teeth? That's because milk and other dairy products are rich in calcium, a mineral that your body needs to make bone. Women especially need enough calcium to prevent osteoporosis. The DV for calcium is 1,000 milligrams, though you can supplement up to 1,200 milligrams, particularly if you don't drink much milk.

Magnesium—Found in molasses, nuts, and spinach, magnesium is a mineral your body needs for healthy nerve and muscle functioning, as well as for developing strong bones. Magnesium is often used to alleviate stress and to prevent coronary artery spasms in people prone to heart attack. The DV is 400 milligrams—a safe supplemental amount.

Phosphorus—Found in meats, fish, poultry, and dairy products, phosphorous is calcium's work mate in helping the body develop strong bones and is sometimes used for tooth and gum problems. The DV for phosphorus is a whopping 1,000 milligrams. There is no need to supplement this mineral, because Americans generally get more than they need from everyday foods.

Potassium—Baked potatoes, bananas, and avocados are super sources of potassium—a mineral that your body needs to maintain vital fluid balances and to help nerves and cells function properly. Potassium is frequently used to help control high blood pressure. The DV is 3,500 milligrams. You should not supplement potassium without asking a doctor.

Sodium—Salt and salty foods are the primary source of sodium. Your body uses sodium to maintain its balance of vital fluids. But don't worry about supplementing this mineral. Americans get more than enough of it in their salty diets. In fact, most doctors recommend that we subtract rather than supplement sodium in our diet. Even so, the DV is 2,400 milligrams.

Zinc—Oysters are supreme sources of this essential mineral, and you can get it from lean meats and other seafood as well. Zinc is a must-have mineral for wound healing, healthy appetite, and sperm production. It is frequently used to speed healing from surgery and to help vitamin C fight colds. The DV for zinc is fifteen milligrams. You can supplement up to thirty milligrams a day, say experts.

Trace Minerals

Regular minerals are found in fairly high concentrations in food. Trace minerals, as the name implies, are found in only minute amounts. Here are several examples.

Chloride—Found in the same salty foods as sodium, chloride is helpful for aiding digestion and for helping sodium in maintaining balance among your body's fluids. There is no DV for chloride and, like sodium, there is no need to supplement this commonly-consumed mineral.

Chromium—Whole grains, cheese, and black pepper are good sources of chromium—a trace mineral your body uses to metabolize carbohydrates. It is frequently used for treating symptoms of diabetes and hypoglycemia. It also appears useful for helping prevent hardening of the arteries. There is no DV for chromium, but experts say you can safely supplement fifty to 200 micrograms a day.

Copper—Found in shellfish and cocoa, copper is necessary for forming blood cells and connective tissue. Copper is sometimes used clinically for treating fatigue and anemia. The DV is two milligrams. Many nutritionists say you should not supplement copper because it interferes with the absorption of zinc and can be toxic in high levels, though taking a multivitamin-mineral supplement containing 100 percent of the DV is generally considered safe.

Fluoride—You can find fluoride in fish, tea, and, of course, fluoridated water. This mineral is well-known for strengthening tooth enamel. And studies indicate that fluoride may also be helpful for preventing osteoporosis. There is no DV for fluoride. Generally experts suggest getting between 1.5 and 4.0 micrograms of fluoride daily. There is no need to take supplements because we drink it daily in our water.

Iodine—Most prevalent in iodized salt, iodine is also found in seafood. Your body needs iodine for your thyroid gland to function properly. Iodine is used to treat goiter—a condition that is caused by iodine deficiency—and some nutritionists believe it can be helpful for preventing osteoporosis. The DV for iodine is 150 micrograms. Most people have no need to supplement iodine. If you're on a low-salt diet, however, you may want to discuss iodine supplementation with your doctor.

Iron—Meats, tofu, and raisins are good sources for iron. Your body needs this trace mineral for your blood to carry oxygen to your muscles, which is why having too little iron is a major culprit behind fatigue. Iron is primarily used to treat iron-deficiency anemia. The DV is just eighteen milligrams. Because too much iron can cause health problems, experts recommend getting more iron from foods, not supplements, though taking a multivitamin-mineral supplement with 100 percent of the DV is okay. To increase your body's absorption of the iron you eat, try eating iron-rich foods along with foods that contain vitamin C, because vitamin C aids in the absorption of iron.

Manganese—Nuts, whole-grain cereals, and tea are some good sources of manganese. This trace mineral is essential for maintaining connective tissue and cellular integrity. It may also prove helpful for treating some of the muscle rigidity associated with Parkinson's disease, though more research is needed to know for sure. There is no DV for manganese, but experts say you can supplement ten to twenty milligrams safely.

Molybdenum—Reach for legumes, meats, and whole-grain cereals for your daily dose of molybdenum—a trace mineral that your body uses to process carbohydrates, to produce uric acid, and to properly use the trace mineral iron. Molybdenum may also help reduce levels of cancer-causing nitrates and nitrites in the body. There is no DV for this trace mineral, as research on it is still in its infancy. Experts say you can supplement about 150 micrograms of molybdenum. You should not supplement molybdenum in amounts higher than 500 micrograms, because it may cause copper loss.

Selenium—Meats, whole-grain cereals, and Brazil nuts are great ways to get more selenium. This trace mineral is an antioxidant and also assists the antioxidant action of vitamin E. Researchers have found that selenium helps prevent cardiovascular disease and cancer. There is no DV for selenium, but experts suggest supplementing between 100 and 200 micrograms a day.

The General Benefits

Aside from the specific benefits of taking specific supplements, researchers have found that just taking a multivitamin and mineral supplement every day can produce enormous improvements in health and well-being.

It's common for problems such as fatigue, forgetfulness, insomnia, and mood swings to lift in response to general vitamin and mineral supplementation, particularly among older adults. And more and more studies are indicating that vitamin and mineral supplementation can help stave off serious degenerative diseases such as heart disease, diabetes, and cancer. How much you can expect to pay depends on the vitamins and minerals you need to take. Supplement prices can range from a few dollars a month to more than a hundred dollars.

Because there is so much information and misinformation surrounding vitamin and mineral supplementation, the best thing you can do for yourself is talk to a medical professional trained in nutritional supplementation. Though an increasing number of mainstream medical doctors are learning the benefits of vitamin and mineral therapy, it generally isn't their forte. Your best bet is to find a naturopathic or holistic medical provider whose training focuses on healing the body with nutritional supplementation.

FOR MORE INFORMATION

Unlike some other alternative health therapies such as chiropractic or aromatherapy, you can't just look up vitamins and minerals in the yellow pages and find a "vitamin and mineral practitioner" in your area. The following organization, however, may help you locate a qualified professional.

American College of Advancement in Medicine
P.O. Box 3427
Laguna Hills, California 92654
714-583-7666

YOGA

An Ancient Twist on Modern Healing

Forget the pictures you've seen of the double-jointed man with his feet crossed behind his head. That has as much to do with yoga as crossing the English Channel has to do with swimming. Despite our contorted images, yoga is nothing more than relaxing and connecting your mind and body.

The word yoga comes from the Sanskrit *yuj*, meaning "to yoke." The purpose of yoga is to yoke—or create unity between—your mind, body, and breathing. This involves deep breathing, gentle stretching, and some quiet meditation. Yoga positions are designed to both strengthen and relax you, while allowing your body's fluids to course smoothly through their channels and replenish your organs and tissues. Ancient texts teach that yoga clears up accumulated stress in the body, which otherwise prevents your body's vital energy, or *prana*, from flowing freely. When prana is obstructed, emotional distress and sickness are the result, yoga practitioners believe.

Of all the alternative therapies, yoga is the simplest, not to mention the least expensive. All you need is about thirty minutes, a quiet space, and a little instruction to reap a host of health benefits, including reducing stress, easing premenstrual and menopausal symptoms, alleviating back pain, preventing cardiovascular disease, lessening asthma attacks, and reducing the symptoms of diabetes.

Take a Deep Breath

The very first yoga move you'll learn is the simplest—and also the most difficult: breathing. Obviously, we breathe all the time. Unfortunately, we don't generally do it right, say yoga experts. Most of us take very shallow breaths, filling up only the top portion of our lungs before we exhale. What we should be doing is what you see babies doing when they breathe—filling our bellies.

To do proper yogic breathing, or *pranayama*, start by sitting comfortably in a chair, with one hand on your stomach. First push the air out of your lungs through your nose. Then relax your stomach muscles and draw a large breath through your nose and into the bottom of your lungs, pushing out your diaphragm. When you're doing it right, the hand on your stomach will go up and down with each breath. You should take about three seconds to inhale and three seconds to exhale.

Though yogic breathing should be part of your daily yoga routine, instructors recommend that you practice deep breathing frequently throughout the day so that it becomes second nature. Yogic breathing by itself is healing in that it relaxes you and provides your body with a better supply of oxygen, say experts. Studies show that, done consistently, pranayama also aids digestion, improves cardiac functioning, and may even reduce the frequency of asthma attacks.

Peaceful Meditation

A couple of thousand years ago, rulers and sages in India used to take to the forests of Northern India to find strength and serenity. There they would consult wise *rishis*, or teachers, on finding inner peace through meditation. The problem was, their bodies were so tight and stressed, they were unable to sit in one position long enough to meditate. The result was *hatha* yoga—the best-known yoga style in the Western world, which uses a balanced program of postures.

171

As is the case with breathing, most experts recommend that you try meditating by itself before you try combining it with yoga poses. The key is relaxing to the point where your mind is completely still.

First, find a quiet, warm room where you can lie down on a mat or a blanket undisturbed. Lie face up with your arms at your sides. Starting at your head, tense and release the muscles in your face, neck, shoulders, arms, and so on, one at a time until you reach your feet. Next, work on quieting your mind. Repeating a mantra, which is a word or sound, for a few minutes can help. The classic yoga mantra is "ohm." Then become silent. You're going to have thoughts, but you want to let them just drift through your mind without dwelling on them. The goal is a completely clear mind. But it's no easy task, so don't be discouraged if you can only manage it for a minute or two on the first try.

YOGA ALERT

As mentioned earlier, people with heart disease or back pain should practice yoga only under the care of their physician. For those who have experienced back problems, a qualified yoga instructor should also be consulted before trying yoga positions.

The ultimate stage of meditation is to reach what is known as *samadhi*, or spiritual realization. This comes after years of practice. It is a state of awareness that is connected to the universe, beyond mind and body.

Strike a Pose

There are literally dozens of positions, or asanas, in yoga that are designed to stretch and strengthen your muscles, improve your posture, and compress and relax your organs and nerves.

Some of the very advanced asanas can be quite challenging. Most, however, are rather simple stretches. Yoga instructors recommend beginning with the easiest poses, and doing several a day until you work up to some that are more difficult. Don't push yourself. Yoga is not a competitive sport.

A few of the best beginner poses to try are the corpse, the half boat pose, and the butterfly, described in the following paragraphs. But to do yoga right, it's best to enroll in a class to learn poses and how to do them correctly. As you progress, you can take more advanced classes. Group classes generally don't cost more than about fifteen dollars a session.

The corpse—Often the first posture you learn, the corpse is also the simplest. Lie on your back with your arms out to the sides about a foot from your body, palms up, and with your feet spread about shoulder-width apart. Close your eyes and breathe using the pranayama technique.

The half boat—Lie flat on your stomach with your forehead touching the floor, your arms straight over your head, your palms touching the floor, and your legs together and straight out. Slowly lift your arms, head, and torso off the floor; hold for five seconds, and lower. Then move your feet about twelve inches apart, keep your legs straight, and slowly lift your legs and feet. Hold for five seconds, and lower.

The butterfly—Sit on the floor or a mat with your back straight. Pull the soles of your feet together and grasp your feet with your hands. Slowly raise and lower your knees so that your legs resemble the wings of a butterfly. Then sit still and gradually lean forward from your hips, keeping your back straight. Hold for a minute. Breathe and lean forward a bit farther. Then return to your original position.

What It Treats

Because of its total body emphasis, from flexibility and strength to breathing and relaxation, yoga is a beneficial treatment or complementary therapy for a host of conditions

173

ranging from asthma to heart disease. The following are some of the areas that have been the most well-documented.

Asthma—Because yoga focuses on controlled, improved breathing, it can be a real boon for people suffering from asthma, say experts. British researchers, for example, found that people suffering from mild asthma experienced improvements in their condition when they practiced *pranayama*, or yogic breathing. Also, they appeared better able to tolerate the effects of histamine—a body chemical that can trigger asthma attacks in people who are sensitive to it.

Diabetes—Another condition that benefits from the stress-relieving aspects of yoga is diabetes. Some medical experts believe that because stress elevates blood sugar, it also aggravates diabetes. Because yoga relieves stress, it can also help keep diabetes in check. Researchers studying 150 people with adult-onset diabetes would agree. They found that when these volunteers with non-insulin-dependent diabetes performed yoga sessions in the morning and in the evening, two out of three showed fair to good improvement on fasting blood sugar and glucose tolerance tests. Many of these subjects were also able to reduce their need for medication significantly.

Heart disease—Because of its role in stress reduction, many alternative and mainstream health practitioners recommend yoga as a way to reduce heart disease risk. Well-known cardiologist Dean Ornish, M.D., incorporates hatha yoga in his program for reversing heart disease. In fact, though walking is an exercise frequently touted for people battling heart disease, researchers have found that certain yoga routines can actually elevate heart rate as effectively as treadmill walking, but without the same taxing metabolic demands. If you already have heart disease, however, it's critical that you ask your doctor to approve any new exercises. You should also get specific training from a certified yoga instructor, to ensure the postures you're using are safe.

Low back pain—Bed rest used to be what the doctor ordered for an aching back. Today, we know that not moving can be the worst thing for back pain. Doctors want to get people moving through their pain, and yoga is one of the key techniques for doing this.

Yoga is useful for strengthening, stretching, and aligning the spine and the back muscles. In one survey of 1,142 people with back pain, 98 percent found yoga beneficial.

Because the back is such a sensitive area, however, it is very important that you consult your doctor or physical therapist, as well as a qualified yoga instructor, before trying any yoga positions to alleviate back pain. Not all positions are designed for people with weak or injured lower backs.

Menopause—Unlike conventional medicine, which treats menopause as a disease that requires hormones, medications, and sometimes even surgery to relieve, alternative medicine practitioners recognize yoga as an ideal treatment for facilitating this important transition in a woman's life. Yoga can help alleviate symptoms of menopause such as hot flashes, vaginal dryness, mood swings, and depression by reducing stress and smoothing out bodily functions.

PMS—As with so many conditions, stress makes premenstrual syndrome worse. By relieving stress, you can often diminish the negative symptoms of PMS, such as cramping and mood swings. Certain passive stretches can also improve circulation in the groin, providing special relief from cramping in that area. Yoga is also considered a form of exercise. And researchers have found that women who exercise for forty-five minutes at least three times a week have decreased premenstrual depression and anxiety compared with women who are sedentary.

Stress-related illness—Of all the areas yoga claims to treat, the one most backed by research is relieving stress. Since yoga started picking up steam in Western countries in the early 1970s, there have been more than 1,000 studies documenting the effectiveness of yoga and meditation for alleviating stress and anxiety. Yoga's goals of achieving inner peace and harmony are helpful for enhancing physical and psychological stamina and health.

As the population ages and people continue to turn to the gentle healing ways of alternative medicine therapies, yoga will likely continue to grow in popularity. Experts in the field recommend that you do it every day to maintain optimum health and balance.

FOR MORE INFORMATION

There are various schools of yoga, and each has its own teaching philosophy. Some are more physical or spiritual than others. You may need to try a few instructors to find the one that matches your needs. The following organizations can help you find the type of yoga and teacher that are right for you.

American Yoga Association
513 S. Orange Avenue
Sarasota, Florida 34236
1-800-226-5859

International Association of Yoga Therapists
109 Hillside Avenue
Mill Valley, California 94941
(Send a self-addressed, stamped envelope for a referral list of teachers in your area.)